The Healthy Families America® Initiative: Integrating Research, Theory and Practice

The Healthy Families America® Initiative: Integrating Research, Theory and Practice has been co-published simultaneously as *Journal of Prevention & Intervention in the Community*, Volume 34, Numbers 1/2 2007.

The Healthy Families America® Initiative: Integrating Research, Theory and Practice

Joseph Galano

Editor

The Healthy Families America® Initiative: Integrating Research, Theory and Practice has been co-published simultaneously as *Journal of Prevention & Intervention in the Community*, Volume 34, Numbers 1/2 2007.

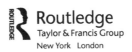

Routledge
Taylor & Francis Group
New York London

First published by The Haworth Press, Inc.

10 Alice Street, Binghamton, N Y 13904-1580

This edition published 2012 by Routledge

Routledge
Taylor & Francis Group
711 Third Avenue
New York, NY 10017

Routledge
Taylor & Francis Group
2 Park Square, Milton Park
Abingdon, Oxon OX14 4RN

The Healthy Families America® Initiative: Integrating Research, Theory and Practice has been co-published simultaneously as *Journal of Prevention & Intervention in the Community,* Volume 34, Numbers 1/2 2007.

The development, preparation, and publication of this work has been undertaken with great care. However, the publisher, employees, editors, and agents of The Haworth Press and all imprints of The Haworth Press, Inc., including The Haworth Medical Press® and Pharmaceutical Products Press®, are not responsible for any errors contained herein or for consequences that may ensue from use of materials or information contained in this work. With regard to case studies, identities and circumstances of individuals discussed herein have been changed to protect confidentiality. Any resemblance to actual persons, living or dead, is entirely coincidental.

The Haworth Press is committed to the dissemination of ideas and information according to the highest standards of intellectual freedom and the free exchange of ideas. Statements made and opinions expressed in this publication do not necessarily reflect the views of the Publisher, Directors, management, or staff of The Haworth Press, Inc., or an endorsement by them.

Library of Congress Cataloging-in-Publication Data

The Healthy Families America Initiative : Integrating Research, Theory and Practice / Joseph Galano, Editor.
       p. cm.
       "Co-published simultaneously as Journal of prevention & intervention in the community, volume 34, numbers 1/2 2007"-T.p. verso.
       Includes bibliographical references and index.
       ISBN 978-0-7890-3680-3 (hard cover) - ISBN 978-0-7890-3681 -0 (soft cover)

       1. Healthy Families America (Project) 2. Family social work-United States. 3. Social work with children-United States. 4. Child abuse-United States-Prevention. I. Galano, Joseph. II. Journal of prevention & intervention in the community.
HV699.H387 2007
362.82'30973-dc22
                                                                                                    2007033147

The Healthy Families America® Initiative: Integrating Research, Theory and Practice

CONTENTS

ABOUT THE EDITOR

Joseph Galano, PhD, is an Associate Professor of Psychology at the College of William and Mary and a core faculty member in the Virginia Consortium Program in Clinical Psychology. He is committed to applying psychology and working directly with communities to address social problems and to improve the human condition. Dr. Galano was awarded Fellow status in the Society for Community Research and Action (APA Division 27). In recognition of his career accomplishments, the American Psychological Association honored him with the 1996 Distinguished Contribution to Practice in Community Psychology award.

Dr. Galano has worked at the local, state, and national levels to prevent child abuse and neglect. He has consulted with Hampton, Virginia's Healthy Families Partnership for over fifteen years. Hampton was twice designated City of the Year for its proactive approach to solving social problems. Since 1995, he has worked with Prevent Child Abuse Virginia to develop Virginia's statewide child abuse prevention initiative, Healthy Families Virginia. He was a member of the steering committee that developed the Blue Ribbon Plan to Prevent Child Abuse and Neglect in Virginia and currently serves on Healthy Families Virginia's Advisory Council. Since 1992 he has been a member of the Healthy Families America (HFA) Research Practice Network and is a member of the HFA State Leaders Network.

His prevention research and advocacy also span some of society's other pressing social issues: perinatal substance abuse, teen pregnancy, and early childhood development. He has served on Virginia's Prevention and Promotion Advisory Council for 25 years and is proud to have helped shape Virginia's three prevention plans. Dr. Galano served as a Williamsburg/James City County Community Action Agency board member and chaired the board for six years. He has worked with Project LINK, a perinatal substance abuse prevention program in six Virginia cities; Square One, a 17-locality partnership recognized by the Annie E. Casey Foundation for its work to ensure that children in Hampton Roads enter kindergarten healthy and ready to learn; and Voices for Virginia's Children and Youth to prepare the "KIDS Count" annual reports on the status of children. He participated in Congressman Robert C.

Scott's Congressional Briefings on Youth Violence and the Congressman's community roundtables with youth.

Dr. Galano's greatest professional satisfaction has been to help prepare the next generation of preventionists. He has helped hundreds of undergraduate and graduate students become involved in community service and public health careers. He was twice nominated for both the President's Award for Service at the College of William and Mary and the Outstanding Faculty Award of the State Council of Higher Education in Virginia.

Introduction:
The Challenge of Integrating Research into Practice

Joseph Galano

College of William & Mary

SUMMARY. The Introduction to this volume on the ways Healthy Families America® (HFA) integrates research, theory, and practice describes nine articles that offer a contemporary snapshot of HFA research and practice, including four empirical articles presenting research and practice at the state, multi-state, or national level and the most comprehensive summary of HFA outcomes. It contrasts the history of child abuse prevention with progress in the fields of substance abuse and violence prevention. It presents arguments underscoring the critical importance of

---

Address correspondence to: Joseph Galano, Department of Psychology, College of William and Mary, P.O. Box 8795, Williamsburg, VA 23187-8795 (E-mail: jxgala@wm.edu).

More people responded to the call for papers than were possible to include. The Editor is grateful to a superb group of reviewers who aided in selecting the manuscripts to be included and whose feedback added significantly to the quality of this volume. Their collective feedback illuminated issues and posed challenges to the authors, adding significantly to the quality of the individual manuscripts and ultimately to the contribution that the book makes to guiding the field. Special thanks must go to Deanna Gomby, who went beyond the call of duty by reviewing every manuscript and providing corrective feedback and valuable insight. Other reviewers were: Julie Chambliss, Claudia Coulton, Anne McDonald Culp, Rex Culp, James Garbarino, Deanna Gomby, Lydia Killos, Jon Korfmacher, Juliette Mackin, Joel Milner, Kristin Moore, Richard Roberts, James Sorensen, Abe Wandersman, and Kate Whitaker.

[Haworth co-indexing entry note]: "Introduction: The Challenge of Integrating Research into Practice." Galano, Joseph. Co-published simultaneously in *Journal of Prevention & Intervention in the Community* (The Haworth Press, Inc.) Vol. 34, No. 1/2, 2007, pp. 1-11; and: *The Healthy Families America® Initiative: Integrating Research, Theory and Practice* (ed: Joseph Galano) The Haworth Press, 2007, pp. 1-11. Single or multiple copies of this article are available for a fee from The Haworth Document Delivery Service [1-800-HAWORTH, 9:00 a.m. - 5:00 p.m. (EST). E-mail address: docdelivery@haworthpress.com].

the researcher-practitioner relationship and the need for an iterative model of action research. It examines implementation and action research challenges, illustrates lessons learned, and recommends ways to strengthen HFA and guide the next phase of child abuse prevention. doi:10.1300/ J005v34n01_01 *[Article copies available for a fee from The Haworth Document Delivery Service: 1-800-HAWORTH. E-mail address: <docdelivery@haworth press.com> Website: <http://www.HaworthPress.com> © 2007 by The Haworth Press, Inc. All rights reserved.]*

KEYWORDS. Healthy Families America, home visitation, child abuse prevention, research to practice

INTRODUCTION

The goal of this volume is to bridge the gaps between research knowledge, professional practice in community-based home visitation, and policy development, highlighting what has been learned about the emerging Healthy Families America (HFA) initiative. The HFA initiative has been driven by the goal of ameliorating the shameful national epidemic of child abuse and neglect. The manuscripts in this collection are about efforts to build and sustain effective HFA home visiting programs in the United States and the lessons learned. This introduction has two goals: to introduce the volume and to call for greater federal leadership and responsibility in child abuse and neglect prevention.

During the last 30 years, the field of child abuse and neglect prevention has taken many new directions with new policies and programs *but too few champions at the national level.* Beginning with the widespread recognition of the "battered child syndrome," there have been important changes in the use of national surveys to assess the incidence and prevalence of child abuse and neglect. There has also been increased documentation of the medical, educational, psychosocial, and economic consequences of abuse. More recent epidemiological research (The ACE Study) has documented the enormous toll that adverse childhood experiences exact, the substantial contribution that adverse childhood experiences make to the 10 leading causes of death and disability in America, and the associated spiraling health care costs (Felitti, 1998). The Centers for Disease Control and Prevention and Kaiser Permanente researchers assert that adverse childhood experiences are the leading determinant of health and well-being in the United States.

Increasing awareness of the national scope of child abuse and neglect along with the dramatic increase in the rate of founded cases created alarm and concern for many child advocacy groups. Encouraged by a Government Accounting Office (1990) review and findings from some of the new prevention approaches, especially the heartening findings of David Olds' Nurse Home Visitation program, the U.S. Advisory Board on Child Abuse and Neglect sounded a call for a national response (U.S. Advisory Board on Child Abuse and Neglect, 1990). Despite the lack of federal leadership and funding, communities felt obligated to act, and a grass-roots community-by-community movement sprang up across the country (sometimes state leadership would follow). This phase of development allowed numerous community agencies to develop partnerships and coalitions (often under the banner of HFA) to spearhead child abuse and prevention efforts. Although this strategy garnered community support resources across a variety of domains during a time of scarcity, it also contributed to an inconsistent understanding of the problem and highly variable approaches to the solution, not an auspicious beginning for HFA.

Contrast HFA's beginning with the ways in which prevention science advanced in the areas of substance abuse and violence prevention. Although much remains to be done in the fields of substance abuse and violence, these scientific domains effectively move from research to practice. HFA must strive to understand and learn from these public health successes. Aided by federal leadership with a clear mission and substantial funding, these two prevention science areas have moved from surveillance and monitoring through several iterations of funded prevention trials. Each iteration has been more sophisticated than the last. Each iteration has moved from an individual intervention focus to increasingly ecological interventions that involve multiple layers and multiple systems. Each iteration has identified specific program models and best practices that have become the building blocks for the next stage of development. Each iteration has added to the theory base that undergirds prevention research and practice and has delineated critical mediators that must be addressed in the next round.

This federal investment has resulted in incredible resources for preventionists, citizens, and policymakers interested in reducing/preventing substance abuse and violence. These included the directory of Model and Promising Prevention Programs, developed under the leadership of Substance Abuse and Mental Health Services Administration (Brounstein, Gardner, & Backer, 2006), "The Red Book" (National Institute on Drug Abuse, 2003), the National Registry of Effective Prevention Programs (Brounstein, Zweig, & Gardner, 1999), and Blueprints Registry of Model Programs (Department of Justice's Office of Juvenile Justice and Delinquency Prevention, 2000). Now that these science-based programs have been developed and made accessible, these federal agencies have increasingly taken on the task of helping states and communities with the challenges associated with widespread dissemination of substance abuse and violence prevention programs.

The field of child abuse and neglect prevention deserves and needs the same strong federal leadership that the fields of substance abuse and violence prevention have received. Building and sustaining effective prevention programs in real world settings may represent the most critical challenge confronting contemporary prevention science.

The articles in this collection deepen our understanding of HFA and contribute to the development and integration of theory, research, and action. The authors represent a wide array of disciplines, agencies, and roles at the local, state, and national levels working together to plan, implement, evaluate, and sustain child abuse and neglect prevention programs. Their collective commitment deserves high praise. Much can be learned from their success and failures. Their reflections on the HFA experience can help to guide the next phase of child abuse and neglect prevention.

This volume focuses on both the HFA Research Network and the national home-visitation initiative. It describes the growth, evolution, and contributions of this research collaborative (50 researchers in 33 states). This book summarizes the historical antecedents and theoretical assumptions that guide the HFA initiative (programs in 38 states in over 450 communities) and presents the most comprehensive summary of emerging outcomes available to date. The volume also examines implementation issues such as fidelity to the program model and local adaptations in the face of complex, shifting, structural challenges; the role of state systems in developing and advocating for sustainable and effective programs; and the analytic, methodological, sociopolitical challenges confronted by community researchers conducting action research. Finally, this work illustrates lessons learned from the last decade, summarizing and making recommendations for policy issues that can strengthen the initiative.

CONTENTS OF THIS VOLUME

The Healthy Families America Initiative: Integrating Research, Theory, and Practice includes nine articles that offer a contemporary snapshot of research and practice in HFA. The intention is to bring together a set of manuscripts that will be meaningful to citizens, practitioners, and policymakers, as well as evaluators and researchers. Four empirical articles present research and practice at the state, multi-state, or national level and the most current comprehensive summary of HFA outcomes to date. The first two articles provide an important historical and national context for understanding both practice and research in HFA.

The contributors of this volume have many years of distinguished contribution to the goals of HFA. They are individuals who value partnerships and who, in the words of Margaret Mead, "Never doubt that a small group of thoughtful, committed citizens can change the world. Indeed, it is the only thing that ever has."

The first article, "Healthy Families America®: Ruminations on Implementing a Home Visitation Program to Prevent Child Maltreatment" by Holton and Harding, provides the reader with a crucial understanding of the history of HFA, HFA's relationship with Prevent Child Abuse America (PCA America), and an insider's view of many of the challenges associated with HFA's rapid ascension (expanding from 25 sites in 1992 to 430 in 2003) as a national prevention initiative. A strength of the article is its frank assessment of implementation challenges, limitations, and external critiques. The authors explain HFA's internal credentialing process and discuss the way the credentialing process contributes to implementation fidelity, concluding with lessons learned and a thoughtful set of recommendations intended to advance existing models of home visiting.

The second article, "Healthy Families America® Research Practice Network: A Unique Partnership to Integrate Prevention Science and Practice" by Galano and Schellenbach, represents the first published account of the history and accomplishments of the HFA Research to Practice Network (RPN). Attempting to integrate researchers and practitioners on this scale is rare. PCA America deserves praise for leadership in attempting to close the elusive research-to-practice gap. The original goal of the RPN was to foster communication among academic researchers, community-based evaluators, and practitioners so as to integrate science-based prevention practices into practice settings. This article provides a rare glimpse inside PCA America's attempt to create a new paradigm of collaboration. The authors acknowledge the limitations of past and current research paradigms in the social and behavioral sciences, especially the tendency to dichotomize research and practice and to devalue "real-world" researchers. The authors describe the evolution of the network from exclusively researchers to researchers and practitioners and the benefits accrued from working together. They examine what was learned about this rare experiment in creating practitioner-scientist partnerships and offer a detailed plan for sustaining and strengthening the RPN in the future.

The next three articles describe HFA's attempt to support state systems development, and two exemplary statewide home visiting programs, Every

Child Succeeds (Ohio and northern Kentucky) and Healthy Families Arizona. Friedman and Schreiber, in their article "Healthy Families America® State Systems Development: An Emerging Practice to Ensure Program Growth and Sustainability," examine HFA's efforts in state systems development in the context of the diffusion of innovation and program replication literature. They consider the research base for their systems approach. The authors describe why having a centralized and efficient infrastructure is critical during an era of fiscal constraints and increased accountability. Benefits of a well-functioning infrastructure include helping states reduce duplication of services, creating economies of scale, coordinating resources, supporting high-quality site development, and promoting the self-sufficiency and growth of community-based programs. The article concludes with the discussion of the state systems benefits and challenges and lessons learned.

The next articles by Ammerman et al., and Krysik and LeCroy deal with the development, implementation, and evaluation of a multi-site and statewide HFA program. Their work is exciting because it is grounded in theory and research but also recognizes the practical constraints and complexities of conducting action-oriented evaluation research in the real-world settings. These evaluations span a 10-year period and provide insights into how researcher-practitioner partnerships mediate program success. Both of these programs developed strong evaluator-practitioner partnerships from the beginning, employed evaluation for quality improvement, and contributed to positive intermediate outcomes, preparing each initiative to go to scale statewide and gradually employ more rigorous evaluation methods. In fact, having well-documented accounts of the evaluation processes that contributed to the development of these statewide initiatives represents a welcome shift away from the exclusive focus on best practices or evidence-based practice as the only path to program improvement. These papers provide a needed corrective, adding to our understanding of how researcher-practitioner relationships may also mediate program successes, just as the doctor-patient relationship is as important as the active ingredients in a pill.

"Development and Implementation of a Quality Assurance Infrastructure in a Multisite Home Visitation Program in Ohio and Kentucky" by Ammerman et al., describes the origins and implementation of Every Child Succeeds, a multi-site home visitation program in southwestern Ohio and northern Kentucky. When home visitation programs go to scale, numerous challenges are faced in implementation and quality assurance. Drawing on models in business and industry, the authors designed a Web-based system (eECS) to optimize quality assurance and generate new learning for the field by systematically collecting and using data to document outcomes and identify clinical needs (such as high levels of maternal depression at enrollment) that can undermine home visitation. They describe the pilot testing of an augmented module to treat depressed mothers, present promising preliminary results, and discuss challenges encountered.

In their article "The Evaluation of Healthy Families Arizona: A Multisite Home Visitation Program," Krysik and LeCroy describe the history of HFAz, tracing its growth from a pilot in two sites in 1991 to 48 sites in urban, rural, and tribal regions of the state by 2004. HFAz is a broadly implemented home visitation program aimed at preventing child abuse and neglect, improving child health and development, and promoting positive parent/child interaction. The authors describe how a unique administrative structure and collaboration between evaluation and quality assurance helped overcome many of the problems familiar to home visitation programs. The evaluation team describes how a systematic focus to improve processes and outcomes has positioned the program for a randomized longitudinal study, highlights key components of the program, and presents encouraging evaluation results.

The final four articles bring together perspectives that are more national or ecological in their scope. The first, "The Promise of Primary Prevention Home Visiting Programs: A Review of Potential Outcomes" by Russell, Britner, and Woolard, reviews the literature on home visiting outcomes. The authors review traditional outcome domains (e.g., child maltreatment, child health, school-readiness) from the literature on HV, as well as nontraditional outcome domains (e.g., community connection, maternal life course, resilience, child/family wellness) that may be relevant for future evaluations. The authors identify some of the key impediments to effectiveness, including program fidelity, client risk level, intensity of services, and the failure to address community and organizational-level risks. They conclude that home visitation is a promising but largely untested service delivery model for strengthening parents and communities and fostering positive developmental outcomes for children. The authors assert that programs that document their implementation and study their outcomes through a thoughtful, planned process may capture important and much needed information on strengthening families through HV.

The second, "Healthy Families America® Effectiveness: A Comprehensive Review of Outcomes" by Harding, Galano, Martin, Huntington, and Schellenbach, describes the most contemporary and comprehensive summary of HFA outcomes to date. Since the inception of HFA, there has been a growing demand for research on its effectiveness. This paper reviews 32 evaluations (distilled from over 100 evaluation reports) of affiliated HFA sites, nearly half of which include a randomized control or comparison group. Outcome domains include child health and development, maternal life course, parenting, and child abuse and neglect. Parenting outcomes (such as parent-child interaction and parenting attitudes) show the most consistent positive impacts. Mixed results in other domains indicate the need for in-depth research to identify key practices in the most successful sites. The authors discuss several factors that may contribute to differences in outcomes, including recent augmentations to program design, and variability in site implementation and quality, and in family risk levels at enrollment. Such variability in implementation presents a challenge for synthesizing results. The paper also includes highlights from two evaluations of programs that have gone to scale, one community-wide (Hampton, Virginia) and one statewide (Indiana), to illustrate the innovative approaches to evaluation found in HFA research. Overall, researcher-practitioner partnerships are found to be a significant strength of HFA.

The final two articles are unusual because they move to the macro level to explain how physical and social aspects of the environment impact child abuse prevention programs and how future solutions must go beyond traditional attempts to fix the individual and embrace more public health approaches. The first, "The Role of Community in Facilitating Service Utilization" by Daro et al., examines the role community characteristics play in influencing a parent's decision to use voluntary child abuse prevention programs. Nine programs serving families in six states were participants. Multiple regression techniques were used to determine if community characteristics, such as neighborhood distress and the community's ratio of caregivers to those in need of care, predict service utilization levels. The authors' findings suggest that certain community characteristics are significant predictors of the extent to which families utilize voluntary family supports. Contrary to the authors' assumptions, however, new parents living in the most disorganized communities received more home visits than program participants living in more organized communities. The authors recommend using community capacity building to improve participant retention. PCA America created the framework for this multi-state collaboration. That collaboration was not an end in itself, but a means to research that is capable of informing us about how to improve child abuse and neglect prevention programs.

The final article, "Potential Lessons from Public Health and Health Promotion for the Prevention of Child Abuse" by Martin, Green, and Gielen, reviewed two of the most successful public health efforts of the last third of the 20th century–tobacco control and automobile injury control–to understand how changes occur and to generalize from those arenas to child abuse and neglect prevention. The article identifies potential lessons for the field of child abuse prevention. The authors distill the lessons learned and provide five specific recommendations for child abuse and neglect prevention professionals: Investigate varied logic models or conceptual frameworks to identify new opportunities for effective intervention; use a multi-disciplinary, multi-sector approach; normalize desired behaviors and denormalize undesirable behaviors; balance efficacy, feasibility, and cultural appropriateness; and develop strategies for effective policy advocacy based upon who benefits and who shoulders most of the burden. The authors conclude with suggestions about how to frame child abuse and neglect prevention to best impact citizens and public policy.

Selecting articles for this volume required difficult choices. Page limitations and the need to avoid redundancy necessitated excluding all site-level submissions and limiting articles about statewide initiatives to two. These two were not chosen because they assured positive outcomes but because of their commitment to the HFA model and to program evaluation, a commitment sustained over a meaningful time span. While these two articles do describe exemplary state initiatives, other excellent state programs are not represented here. For instance, the HFA site in New York was recently recognized as a "program that works" by the Rand Corporation (Mitchell-Herzfeld, Izzo, Greene, Lee, & Lowenfels, 2005). The time required to provide documentation for this recognition precluded the site from submitting an article for this collection. The New York HFA is committed to continuing its rigorous evaluation, and it promises to offer meaningful contributions to the field of child abuse prevention.

Another statewide initiative that is not discussed in this volume is Alaska's. In June of 2006, the funding for Healthy Families Alaska (HFAK) ended. A recent Johns Hopkins randomized trial (Duggan, in press) determined that although HFAK was not effective in preventing child abuse and neglect, it did produce positive impacts in four critical child and family domains. Moreover, the researchers identified areas to target for improvement and the program had already instituted some of those recommendations. The Johns Hopkins team recommended continuing to provide services to these high risk families. However, the Alaska legislature decided to end funding for the program. The February 20, 2006 newspaper headline in the *Anchorage Daily News* read: "Funding ends for Healthy Families program: Program to prevent child abuse and neglect not effective, state says." During a PCA America sponsored conference call with participants from nearly forty states, I asked the Johns Hopkins research team if an equally fair headline would have been, "Study finds encouraging results in four critical domains, but not in the area of preventing child abuse and neglect." They agreed. Importantly, the assessed levels of risk for these Alaska families as measured by the KEMPE scale (Korfmacher, 2000) at enrollment, as well as women's entry levels of domestic violence, maternal depression, and substance abuse, were the highest of any HFA program to date.

The Alaska project represents a missed opportunity. The *sine qua non* of prevention science is the implementation of effective, enduring programs in real communities. A state facing a major social problem was receiving the expertise of a talented team of researchers who were engaged in the reiterative process of program design, evaluation, and feedback leading to modification. Instead of following this schema, eloquently articulated by Donald Campbell (Campbell, 1991), the Alaska legislature cut funding. Thus, it abandoned the process just as HFAK was moving into the next phase of improving services to some of the highest risk families in the nation. In addition to the disservice to the Alaskan families, this premature action denies prevention scientists the opportunity to learn how to protect children and families who face more than their share of adversity.

What happened in Alaska epitomizes the challenge facing researchers who want to conduct scientific, ethical evaluations. Seeing programs de-funded tempts program managers and state leaders to present only the most favorable findings or to re-analyze data until favorable results can be produced, instead of reporting accurately on scientific, ethical research. The Alaska experience confirms the worst fears of program managers, state leaders, and advocates: that research evaluation results can and will be used against a program, instead of being used to improve it.

REFERENCES

Brounstein, P. J., Gardner, S., & Backer, T. (in press). Moving effective prevention to scale. In P. Tolan, J. Scazpoznik, & S. Sambrano (Eds.), *Improving life trajectories: An assessment of CSAP's predictor variable multi-site study*. Washington, DC: American Psychological Association Press.

Brounstein, P. J., Gardner, S. E., & Backer, T. E. (2006). Research to practice: Efforts to bring effective prevention to every community. *Journal of Primary Prevention, 27,* 91-109.

Brounstein, P. J., Zweig, J. M., & Gardner, S. (1999). *Understanding substance abuse prevention toward the 21st century: A primer on effective programs* [CSAP Technical Report, DHHS Publication No. SMA 99-3301]. Washington, DC: US Government Printing Office.

Campbell, D. T. (1991). Methods for the Experimenting Society. *Evaluation Practice,* *12*(3): 223-260.

Demer, L. (2006, February 20). Funding ends for Healthy Families program: Program to prevent child abuse and neglect not effective, state says. *Anchorage Daily News,* p. B1.

Department of Justice, Office of Juvenile Justice and Delinquency Prevention (2000). *Blueprints for violence prevention* [Publication Number NCJ 204274]. Washington, DC: Department of Justice, Office of Juvenile Justice and Delinquency Program.

Duggan, A., Caldera, D., Rodriguez, K., Burrell, L., Rohde, C., Shea, S. (In press). Impact of a Statewide Home Visiting Program to Prevent Child Abuse. *Child Abuse & Neglect.*

Felitti, V. J., Anda, R. F., Nordenberg D., Williamson, D. F., Spitz A. M., Edwards V. et al. (1998). *Relationship of childhood abuse and household dysfunction to many of the leading causes of death in adults.* The Adverse Childhood Experiences (ACE) study. American Journal of Preventive Medicine.

Government Accounting Office (GAO) (1990). *Home Visiting: A promising early intervention strategy for at-risk families* (GAO/HRD-90-83). Washington, DC: Author.

Korfmacher, J. (2000). The Kempe Family Stress Inventory: A review. *Child Abuse and Neglect, 24*:129-140.

Mitchell-Herzfeld, S., Izzo, C., Greene, R., Lee, E., & Lowenfels, A. (2005). Evaluation of Healthy Families New York (HFNY): First year program impacts. Rensselaer, NY: New York State Office of Children and Family Services, Bureau of Evaluation and Research, Albany, NY: Center for Human Services Research, University at Albany.

National Institute on Drug Abuse (2003). *Preventing drug use among children and adolescents* [NIH Publication Number 04-4212]. Washington, DC: National Institute on Drug Abuse.

U.S. Advisory Board on Child Abuse and Neglect (1990). *Child abuse and neglect: Critical first steps in responding to a national emergency* (Report 3rd). Washington, DC: U.S. Department of Health and Human Services, US Government Printing Office.

doi:10.1300/J005v34n01_01

Healthy Families America®: Ruminations on Implementing a Home Visitation Program to Prevent Child Maltreatment

John K. Holton
Kathryn Harding

Prevent Child Abuse America

SUMMARY. Following a 1990 federal report forecasting a national child abuse and neglect epidemic, Prevent Child Abuse America (PCA America) promoted a home visitation program known as Healthy Families America (HFA). HFA achieved rapid adoption and implementation across the nation going from 25 sites in 1992 to 430 in a decade. In this article, the authors describe PCA America's approach to develop, promote, oversee, and evaluate a national home visitation program. Despite its promising growth, HFA has been criticized for failing to achieve the goal of preventing child maltreatment. HFA's past and present are critiqued based on theory and implementation practice of home visitation and its future projected from the perspective of insiders. Developing a better understanding of HFA's history will advance existing models of home visitation and add to the emerging knowledge base of child maltreatment prevention. doi:10.1300/J005v34n01_02 [Article copies available for a fee from The Haworth Document Delivery Service:

Address correspondence to: John K. Holton, Prevent Child Abuse America, 500 North Michigan Avenue, Chicago, IL 60611.

[Haworth co-indexing entry note]: "Healthy Families America®: Ruminations on Implementing a Home Visitation Program to Prevent Child Maltreatment." Holton, John K., and Kathryn Harding. Co-published simultaneously in *Journal of Prevention & Intervention in the Community* (The Haworth Press, Inc.) Vol. 34, No.1/2, 2007. pp. 13-38; and: *The Healthy Families America® Initiative: Integrating Research, Theory and Practice* (ed: Joseph Galano) The Haworth Press, 2007, pp. 13-38. Single or multiple copies of this article are available for a fee from The Haworth Document Delivery Service [1-800-HAWORTH, 9:00 a.m. - 5:00 p.m. (EST). E-mail address: docdelivery@haworthpress.com].

1-800-HAWORTH. E-mail address: <docdelivery@haworthpress.com> Website: <http://www.HaworthPress.com> © 2007 by The Haworth Press, Inc. All rights reserved.]

KEYWORDS. Child abuse prevention, home visitation, Healthy Families America

The Secretary of Health and Human Services, in conjunction with his counterparts in the Federal Government . . . and the Governors of the several states should ensure that efforts to prevent the maltreatment of children are substantially increased. Such efforts, at a minimum, should involve a significant expansion in the availability of home visitation and follow-up services for all families of newborns.

(US DHHS, Advisory Board on Child Abuse and Neglect, 1990)

THE BEGINNING:
FROM HEALTHY START TO HEALTHY FAMILIES

In the final decade of the 20th century, the U.S. Advisory Board on Child Abuse and Neglect issued a report calling for immediate and urgent attention directed at the "national emergency" of child abuse in the United States. A second report concentrated its recommendations on the federal government's role and strongly emphasized the importance of making prevention a key strategy by implementing a voluntary, universal neonatal home visitation program (US DHHS, 1991). As child abuse remains a magnet for news attention, the advisory report warnings and its call to action made national headlines. One organization, the National Committee to Prevent Child Abuse (NCPCA), currently known as Prevent Child Abuse America (PCA America), decided to change the way it conducted business and sought to put in place one of the several recommendations put forth by the advisory body. In looking at the existing models for home visitation, a key recommendation to prevent child maltreatment, PCA America decided to begin its efforts based on a model found literally in the "middle of the ocean." The purpose of this article is to tell the story of Healthy Families America (HFA), PCA America's home visitation model, from the inside-out, describing the program's beginnings, present, and projected future. In doing so, the article explains the current model of HFA and put forth lessons learned with the hope that preventionists in fields serving children will benefit from this experience and move the country closer to the goal of ending the epidemic of abuse and neglect.

HFA owes its beginnings to several sources, none more important than the Hawaii Family Stress Center, which instituted a home visitation service envisioned by C. Henry Kempe, the pediatrician often credited with identifying child abuse as a social problem. In their widely influential publication, Kempe et al. (1962) did two things: firstly, it disqualified, or at least held suspect, caregiver explanations for children's injuries such as subdural and retina bleeding, contusions, broken bones, or burns offered to medical personnel; and secondly, it marked the medical community's commencement to address systematic injuries to children. Kempe argued that parents were the key to prevention. To support parents, particularly those in need, Kempe developed an assessment tool (Kempe & Kempe, 1976; Korfmacher, 2000; Orkow, 1985) to guide home visits by a well-trained and supervised staff (Kempe, 1976a). The Hawaii Family Stress Center further developed Kempe's approach which resulted in "Healthy Start," a home visitation program initiated in 1975. In time the practice spread across the state and by the early 1980s had come to the attention of mainland states (see Appendix 1, "A Short History of the Hawaii Family Stress Center").

Another home visiting model focusing on the health needs of new mothers, the Prenatal/Early Intervention Project, P/EIP,[1] began in Elmira, New York as a health promotion and smoking cessation randomized experiment (Olds, Henderson, Chamberlin, & Tatelbaum, 1986). In addition to improvements in maternal health and life course activities, P/EIP brought scientific evidence to bear in support of home visiting as an efficacious approach to prevent child maltreatment. Both Healthy Start and P/EIP programs achieved national stature when the Advisory Board highlighted the importance of parents starting their child rearing journey with support, guidance, and knowledge. Preventing child abuse and neglect, as stressed by Dr. Kempe and detailed in the Advisory Board's report, begins with good parenting and continues with good community support (Kempe, 1976b).

Up to the 1990 Advisory Board report, federal efforts to prevent child maltreatment were legislated by the Child Abuse Prevention and Treatment Act (CAPTA), created by Congress in 1974. Funding from CAPTA created the National Center on Child Abuse and Neglect or *NCCAN* (now *OCAN*—the Office on Child Abuse and Neglect) and supported state legislative efforts to define what could be considered child maltreatment and to develop the necessary infrastructure for intervention and remediation. As authorized and funded by CAPTA, states designed protocols to intervene in the lives of families as warranted. Although, NCCAN sponsored periodic national conferences, research, and occasionally, demonstration prevention programs, no prevention program had been promulgated for the nation, however, and the existing research/program undertakings were limited by the brevity of federal funding cycles. Reducing child maltreatment in this manner would waste generations of children, PCA America argued, given the professional community's historical obstinacy to acknowledge child maltreatment and societal reluctance to challenge sacrosanct values that deem children parental property (Golden, 1992; Nelson, 1984; Roberts, 2002).

During the intervening years between legislating CAPTA and the Advisory Board report, the rise in public awareness of child maltreatment corresponded to the escalation of reports of abuse and neglect (Daro, 1998, 1999). The Advisory Board's "national warning" (US DHHS, Advisory Board on Child Abuse and Neglect, 1990) of the child maltreatment epidemic responded to public concerns and called for an action agenda. The Advisory Board criticized the status quo federal strategy of funding "discretionary programs" as a means of accumulating knowledge. To address this national epidemic and promote the merits of prevention to reduce the numbers of abused children, PCA America endorsed the Advisory Board recommendations and the idea of universal home visiting. Encouraged by the interest of several states to implement prevention programs coupled with the promising results from the Olds et al. (1986) home visitation program, PCA America took steps to promote a model fashioned after Healthy Start. With financial support from the Ronald McDonald's House Charities, PCA America collaborated with the Hawaii Family Stress Center to introduce home visitation services for new parents to the rest of the country as "Healthy Families America" (HFA). Naming PCA America's home visitation program, "Healthy Families America" was due to the use of "Healthy Start" by wellness efforts linked to infant mortality reduction, heart disease prevention, and other health concerns.

Making the decision to promote home visitation was in keeping with the prevention approaches detailed years earlier by PCA America's executive director, Anne Cohn Donnelly:

> Based on what is known or believed to enhance an individual's ability to function in a healthy way within a family . . . a strategy for prevention [includes:] (a) support programs for new parents, (b) education for parents, (c) early and regular child and family

screening and treatment, (d) child care opportunities, (e) programs for abused children and young adults, (f) life skills training for children and young adults, (g) self-help groups and other neighborhood supports and (h) family support services. (1983, p. 25)

Previously, PCA America's national efforts to promote prevention via public awareness, advocacy, research, and capacity building through a network of local chapters had encompassed many different approaches to reduce child maltreatment; now it would push for a singular focus.

News of this decision was not received enthusiastically by all PCA America staff and chapters as it meant other promising prevention strategies already underway could not be nurtured to maturity. Several chapters, for example, had developed curricula and were training educators, law enforcement, legal and court personnel, and other professionals on child maltreatment and its prevention. The PCA-Georgia chapter had begun a large-scale initiative to provide new parents with linkage and referral services needed in the first year of the child's life. Efforts of prevention initiatives among other chapters, such as legislation to prevent corporal punishment in schools or the development of child sexual abuse prevention programs, were growing.

Given the decision to focus PCA America resources, several questions had to be addressed simultaneously, beginning with how a national nonprofit organization could introduce, promote, and sustain a program to be implemented at the local level. PCA America responded by creating expert teams or panels to advise HFA's development. The initial teams who traveled to Hawaii to observe Healthy Start firsthand were state leaders representing interested and influential staff from local and state departments of public health and child welfare, as well as PCA America chapter leaders. A second panel consisted of Hawaii Family Stress Center consultants, PCA America's internal national trainers, and technical assistance authorities borrowed from institutions known for their expertise in training practitioners in complex tasks. A third panel was comprised of researchers interested in studying home visiting and evaluating HFA, and was brought together under the auspices of the National Center for Child Abuse Prevention Research (National Center). The National Center had conducted the first randomized control study of Healthy Start, validating some of the earlier claims of effectiveness in preventing maltreatment and fostering child well-being (Daro, McCurdy, & Harding, 1998). To expedite knowledge exchange to enhance practice, the National Center formalized a Research Network on Home Visiting with funding from the Carnegie Corporation. Local evaluation efforts were initiated nearly as quickly as site implementations. See Black et al. (2000) as an early example. Collectively, the three panels of state leaders, trainers, and evaluators would lay the foundation for implementing the new initiative. HFA would be a home visitation program with three goals: improving child health, improving parenting effectiveness, and preventing child abuse and neglect. For the purposes of launching HFA, organizing political will, assembling expert teams, and articulating goals were necessary starting points; implementing a national initiative would require much more, beginning with theoretical guidance.

IMPLEMENTATION: MOVING FROM THEORIES TO PRACTICE

Given the complexity of preventing child maltreatment, HFA would need more than one theoretical approach. The causes or "risk factors" for maltreatment often are related to a variety of caregiver and familial behaviors or circumstances. In addition, external conditions aggravated by levels of income and literacy impoverishment, crime, scarcity of services, or influences stemming from community disorganization all contribute to the type and frequency of child maltreatment. Selecting which risk factors to mitigate presumes a capability to predict the likelihood of injury *to whom, by whom*. HFA, therefore, aimed its prevention goals at new parents facing familial and community stressors. As implemented, HFA would change caregiving behaviors so as to remove parental risk factors from the maltreatment equation. Secondarily, by working in concert with communities desiring HFA, alliances and collaborations among agencies within the community would develop to promote continuous support for the newborn's first 5 years of life. Compatible individual, family, and community change theories were examined, beginning with the targeted population–new parents.

Achieving the goal specific to child maltreatment prevention would depend in part on changing individual behaviors, specifically those which reduce caregiver risks or enhance protective factors. For example, parents who possess protective factors for child well-being, notably psychosocial readiness, knowledge and competence, are less likely to maltreat their children (Schumaker, Smith Slep, & Heyman, 2001; Harrington & Dubowitz, 1999; Egeland, Sroufe, & Erikson, 1983). Psychological theories of attachment (Bowlby, 1988; Bowlby, Ainsworth, Boston, & Rosenbluth, 1956) informed the goal of improving parenting skills, and social learning theory (Bandura, 1971) provided the conceptual framework for doing so in a non-laboratory setting. However, keeping to its roots in prevention programming, PCA America would anchor HFA's prevention rationale in social ecology.

Ecology examines behavior broadly, taking into consideration as much of the surrounding "context" as possible. Ecologic analyses of complex behaviors such as child abuse go beyond the immediate victim-perpetrator dyad. Promoting prevention requires an understanding of roles to be played by caregivers, family, institutions, neighborhood, and society at-large (Belsky, 1980; Bronfenbrenner, 1977; Cicchetti & Lynch, 1993; Garbarino & Barry, 1997). Moreover, embracing ecology theory underscored a departure from other prevention approaches that identified child maltreatment as an exclusive domain of individual or family dysfunction (Daro & Donnelly, 2003). The ecological approach to understanding child abuse takes into account an individual's responses to other persons, events, and environmental factors and their interactions (Maas, 1975). Ecologic hypotheses state that within a given community, risk factors for child maltreatment can be neutralized and protective factors can be augmented (Oates, 1982). Garbarino and Barry (1997) suggest that community features can magnify or minimize parental weaknesses. Brooks-Gunn (1995) found community social assets could serve to reinforce parental strengths as did the Molnar et al. (2003) investigation of community differences in use of corporal punishment. In addition, acknowledging the importance of devising a strategy of removing or reducing risks located in the broader, macro-environment outside the family (Azar, Povilaitis, Lauretti, & Pouquette, 1998; Trickett & Shellenbach, 1998) led HFA to public health theories. Public health starts with prevention instead of intervention or treatment.

Conceptually, public health views illness and injury prevention as keys to health and well-being (Green & Kreuter, 2004). Public health research applications typically employ a multi-level approach to prevention that starts with data collection (surveillance) to identify risk and protective factors; intervention(s) follow and the results are evaluated and disseminated (US Department of Health and Human Services, 2000). Treating child maltreatment prevention as a public health issue established the link between abuse and future health-related problems, described in considerable depth by Felitti et al. (1998) and others (Hammond, 2003). Theoretical guidance of HFA resulted in an acknowledgment of the child's environment with an emphasis on reducing risk at both individual (caregiver) and community (social services) levels. The next task was to put theory into action, particularly since HFA services on the continental United States were to be deployed among more heterogeneous populations, neighborhoods, and providers.

HFA put forth 12 critical elements as an ensemble of services deemed necessary to create safe, nurturing, and healthy experiences for children. The critical elements were gleaned from research literatures relative to "best practices" of home visiting (see Appendix 2–HFA's Critical Elements). Enhancing the perinatal and postnatal attachment experiences for parent and child, increasing parental self-efficacy to access and utilize community resources and services, and modeling and supporting parental self-care, autonomy, and skills development comprise the critical elements (Guterman, 2001; Harding, 2002). The challenge of answering the "why" of HFA was addressed by theories; answering the implementation questions of "what," "whom," "when," "where," and "how" were encapsulated within the critical elements' three areas of (a) service initiation, accessibility, and continuity; (b) service content; and, (c) staff characteristics and supervision.

Concerns about maintaining model fidelity emerged after the initial cohort of HFA staffs was trained and services had commenced. If HFA allowed for site-specific adaptations to meet the diversity of participants, staff, and administering organizations, states insisted that an overarching quality assurance system be instituted to standardize implementation. PCA America approached the Council on Accreditation of Services for Children and Families (COA) for assistance, and a partnership to assist HFA sites in meeting the demands of credentialing was secured. The process of standardizing HFA programs was developed in 1995, piloted in 1996, and instituted in 1997 as "credentialing" (*Healthy Families Credentialing Manual*, 1999). The credentialing purpose was twofold: (a) determine the extent to which an HFA program adhered to the critical elements and, (b) provide organizations who implemented the model with fidelity with the HFA seal of approval. The credentialing process involves a guided, extensive self-assessment review, followed by an independent peer-lead site visit (see Appendix 3–HFA Credentialing Example).

Credentialed programs maintain use of the HFA name, logo, and HFA affiliation, and they are eligible for joint grant and knowledge-building opportunities with PCA America. Healthy Families program staff can network with peers from other credentialed programs, work with other members to shape the direction of the initiative, take advantage of national and state level advocacy for HFA services, coordinate training and technical assistance, and partner in public awareness efforts. As an enticement for becoming credentialed, a time-intensive process that often extends a full year or more, program sites have access to technical assistance from PCA America and to HFA materials at a reduced cost or free of charge. PCA America moved to decentralize its training and technical assistance role by creating Regional Resource Centers (RRCs) for future credentialing of HFAs. Ideally, RRCs will be geographically located to provide requested services formerly provided by PCA America national office staff or its consultants. The decentralization move is in keeping with PCA America's approach of empowering local capacity, replicating the organization's state chapter network.

THE PRESENT:
HFA UNDER THE MICROSCOPE

Questions regarding the efficacy of home visiting programs, including HFA and its ability to achieve expected outcomes, were detailed in the Packard Foundation's *The Future of Children* (1999). The issue focused on evaluations of home visiting programs and suggested that the modest findings for preventing maltreatment were both unanticipated and disappointing given earlier predictions of efficacy by Foundation staff (Sherwood, 2005). Although acknowledging that the complex challenges facing home-based services contributed to the mixed outcomes, Gomby et al. (1999) argued for "a dedicated effort, led by the field, to improve the quality and implementation of existing home visiting services" (p. 24). A few years later, uncertainty about home visiting as a preventive approach to maltreatment was reignited by a Task Force report to the Centers for Disease Control and Prevention (2003) that found home visitation programs in general to be an effective preventive service. Sherwood (2005) offers a critique on the process by Gomby et al., that may have minimized the criticism of home visiting as a prevention program. Nonetheless, questions specific to HFA's effectiveness as a child maltreatment prevention program continue as a number of recent studies note limited, if any, effects (Duggan et al., 2004; Landsverk et al., 2002). Understanding HFA's shortcomings in preventing child maltreatment requires not only examining its quality as implemented but also reassessing its theories guiding its practices of home visitation.

The HFA application of ecological theory broadened the inclusion of maltreatment risks in a child's environment. The problem of child abuse and neglect is understood better (and prevented more effectively) when the risks for its occurrence take into consideration caregiver and community threats. As noted in the National Research Council report (1993), prevention of maltreatment is based on reducing known risks and increasing protective factors. Unraveling child maltreatment begins with acknowledging the multiple components from caregivers, other family members, neighborhoods, and the larger society. Ignoring external influences on behavior, particularly that of other adults and neighbors, may lead to overestimating the ability of individuals to change their behaviors as Coulton et al. (1995) and Sampson et al. (1997) reported. Children living at or below federal poverty guidelines, for instance, face a probability of reported abuse that is nearly 25 times more likely than children living out of poverty (US DHHS, 1996). Unfortunately, ecology theory does not explain whether the condition of poverty is the culprit or whether the occupants of the condition are faulty. Since conditions are more difficult to change than individuals, HFA placed its emphasis on the latter. Helping parents and caregivers change their behavioral risks to a newborn has necessitated adding techniques to support HFA families.[2]

Attachment theory and social learning theory remain integral to HFA practice, but other psychological approaches have been added or adopted to better address other needs. Co-occurring behaviors within families necessitated that HFA programs train staffs in the principles of cognitive behavioral therapy, motivational interviewing, and multi-systemic therapy as a means to gain entrée and guide service delivery with families. Other curricula were selected as well, often addressing the needs of fathers and prenatal parents. One of the challenges HFA programs faced was to find intervention modalities that were compatible with HFA's ecologic orientation and its critical elements practice. The interventions would have to share additional commonalities as well–each approach could readily be adapted to meet the needs of both staff and family participants; each approach would seek to give families "agency," that is, making families "partners" in the change process; each modality had to have an established clinical record and/or be supported by scientific evidence; and each would result in favorable program trends, such as longer retention trajectories for participants and fewer turnovers among staff. As programs sought additional support, the HFA model changed. Today's practice of HFA differs considerably from that of its first model, reflecting the needs of its participating families and raising questions about the viability of its original practice platform.

Today, since every HFA site must implement 12 Critical Elements (see Appendix 2), a review of the credentialing process that HFA uses to foster and ensure implementation fidelity is in order. HFA sites generally support the credentialing process as a way of ascertaining whether quality standards for home visitation are being implemented. Sites disagree whether credentialing leads to an improvement in program operations and participant outcomes. For example, sites have questioned the efficacy of weekly home visits and other "best practices" that lack confirmatory empirical evidence. Systemic incorporation of evaluation findings as a means of replicating successes or changing the practice of HFA has yet to be implemented, thereby limiting generalization of successful programs. Questions also have been raised that challenge the sustainability of the credentialing process when weighed against its cost in time and resources to complete. A few sites chose to devise other methods of assuring quality, thereby losing the HFA name and their ability to continue to participate as a "credentialed program."

In part, the unanticipated national response to HFA, increasing within the first 5 years from a few sites to over 300 communities in 40 states, explains PCA America's inability to closely monitor its prevention product. The other part of the story, ironically, that which is responsible for program monitoring, is shared partly by two components within HFA–its research network and state systems.

Two years after PCA America commenced HFA, the Carnegie Corporation helped fund the HFA Research Network in 1994. The initial aim of the Network was to support HFA by building research and evaluative findings into the model, thus structuring refinements of its underlying assumptions and implementation, and advancing a quality assurance system. To achieve its aims meant the research network would put in place a means of collecting and examining data detailing program operations and outcomes (Partnership Guide, 1998). Receiving, organizing, and synthesizing data has not been as easy as requesting it, however. No single set of reasons, but rather an assortment of events curtailed systematic data gathering nationally from HFA sites. For example, the governmental Health Insurance Portability and Accountability Act (HIPAA) introduced a set of requirements for sharing participant information unforeseen when HFA began. One state legislature issued a decree specific to HFA, prohibiting out-of-state access regardless of whether HIPAA assurances were met; other delays or denials for data sharing were linked to under-funded evaluation budgets (the norm), and incompatible or competing software systems which inhibit data sharing.

Years passed before a grant from the Packard and Gerber Foundations would be secured to build a facilitated dialogue between HFA researchers and practitioners. Positive results included sharing problems and solutions when conducting evaluations as well as sharing research findings and their implications. Thanks to the open and frank discussion of outcomes and program challenges within the Researcher-Practitioner Network, it became clear that implementation issues, such as lower than expected rates of family engagement and retention, were affecting outcomes. In addition, this process of knowledge exchange plays a central role in understanding the need for enhanced program strategies to address the most severe risk factors associated with child maltreatment, including depression, substance abuse, and domestic violence. Intimate partner violence has been identified as one specific domestic problem that can disrupt and attenuate home visiting outcomes (Eckenrode, Ganzel, Henderson, Smith, Olds, Powers et al., 2000). In the interim, Harding et al. (2004) found in a multi-state study of HFA implementation that there were substantial site variations in family risk levels and that that variability contributed to inconsistent outcomes across sites. The significant finding is the lack of generalizability of research beyond specific site programs, a finding raised by others concerned with the spotty evidence of efficacy for HFA recipients (Chaffin, 2004, 2005).

Oversight of HFA by its credentialing process has revealed additional challenges to implementation fidelity. In terms of screening, each program defines its target population based on the needs of its community, resulting in a variation of participants among programs across the country. Most programs enroll a broad range of families, including first-time parents, single parents, teen parents, and parents eligible for public assistance (TANF). The elasticity of intake decisions for HFA participants places greater demands on home visitors and their supervision. Implementing the HFA model depends on the savvy and sophistication of its home visiting staff. Home visits were to be done by a trained and supervised staff who recreate the familial and cultural supports that were provided for in previous generations by extended family members–grandparents, uncles, aunts, cousins and fictive kin. Staffs have two major responsibilities: (a) make a connection with the principal caregiver, and (b) provide the caregiver, most often a first-time parent or young parent under the age of 25, with support typically focused on attachment to the infant and on child development. Home visitors are also responsible for helping families develop realistic plans to meet agreed-upon objectives and assisting the parents to identify and access resources in their own community.

HFA promotion of a staffing model that emphasizes personal characteristics and community experiences is often misinterpreted to mean that all HFA home visitors are paraprofessionals who possess no college or professional education related to conducting visitations (Chaffin & Friedrich, 2004; Olds et al., 2004). As Kempe (1976a) and others have suggested, PCA America's support of paraprofessional staff as home visitors has efficacy evidence (Guterman, 2001; Mendoza, Katz, Robertson, & Rothenberg, 2003; Wasik & Bryant, 2001). While many home visitors come from similar experiences and expectant trajectories for success in life as HFA participants, three-quarters of HFA home visitors, called "Family Support Workers," have attended undergraduate institutions, and many have training in child development (20%) and/or social work (14%) or other relevant areas

(Harding, Friedman, & Diaz, 2003). Their commonalities with HFA participants are believed to facilitate empathy, but unfortunately, they also constitute a level of risk for home visitors to experience the same problems with which they seek to assist program participants (Leventhal, 2004). HFA relies on training and supervision of its home visitors, who in turn, are expected to analyze, synthesize, and evaluate information given to them by the parents. The application of these practice skills (meshed with their real world experiences) contributes to more skillful recruitment, engagement, modeling, imparting of individual and family support, and referrals for other services. Ultimately, the home visitor has to be accepted as a helping agent before benefits to parents commence. Moreover, the list of challenges facing parents and their HFA home visitor reveals the difficulty of problem-solving exacerbated by a caseload population that varies by age, experience, or expectations. In addition, each home visitor may tend to specialize in just one or a few issues or may be unprepared or timorous, addressing family or parenting dysfunction. An example of the latter was found in a recent study that reported HFA home visitors tended to avoid, ignore, or miss altogether family issues with alcoholism and substance abuse, maternal depression, and intimate partner violence (Duggan et al., 2004). It is a finding not limited to HFA or other types of interventions targeted in the home. Previous evidence from other fields suggests that "seasoned" clinical social workers and therapists rarely assess the presence of domestic violence correctly, and even if they do, they are still not likely to intervene effectively (Harway & Hansen, 1993; Harway, 2000; Johnson & Lebow, 2000). HFA, as other programs with a broad approach to family support, may have a difficult time achieving outcomes consistently in the select few areas routinely addressed in outcome evaluation.

HFA does not specify a curriculum that must be used by all home visitors. The choice of curriculum is the decision of the sponsoring agency, and most sites rely on multiple curricula such as *Parents as Teachers* and *MELD*, mixing and matching specific sections to fit a given family. As curricula vary in terms of focus on particular goals such as child development vs. parent-child interaction, the choice of curricula will certainly influence program outcomes; yet the systematic study of curricula used in HFA with regard to comparability of outcomes is in its earliest stages. Nonetheless, a growing interest in research on credentialing is helping HFA understand ways to increase professional and skill development opportunities for staff (Kessler, 2004).

Even if programs conscientiously work to match their selected curricula to HFA goals, there are gaps in what the critical elements address, including the intersection of services received and delivered based on class, race, culture, and language. A frequent critique of the HFA critical elements concerns the lack of specificity on cultural competence, notably the lack of an empirical definition of culturally appropriate materials. Having bilingual staff and translated materials does not ensure cultural competence and falls far short of addressing issues such as structural racism in service delivery and service content. The field of child abuse prevention has not yet provided leadership for practitioners nor empirical research that can guide action (Aspen Institute, 2004; Derezotes, Poertner, & Testa, 2005; Lane et al., 2002; Marable, 2001; Sidelinger et al., 2005).

THE FUTURE FOR HFA

> Neighborhood-based initiatives in poor neighborhoods have always been forced to struggle with the individual and local consequences of national problems whose causes lay outside their purview. They have been shaped by, and at the same time been asked to reconcile, the discrepancy between American ideals and American social realities. (Halpern, 1995)

Universal home visiting for new parents was a key recommendation put forth by the 1990 Advisory Board to tackle the "national emergency" of child maltreatment. It is likely that this key recommendation of home visiting would have been left to languish and never considered for national replication had not PCA America taken steps to avail HFA to scores of interested audiences. In the absence of federal funding, and with no clear signal that prevention of child maltreatment was to become a national public health goal, PCA America responded with a model to promote the wellness of children and prevent their maltreatment. A decade later, much has been learned about the implementation of HFA.[3]

PCA America's investment in HFA is unlike any in its prevention history. Working alongside its chapters and community organizations in social services, child welfare, public health and/or maternal and child health, as well as not-for-profit organizations, HFA's national reach is considerable. Since HFA began, it has provided free home visitation services on a voluntary basis to tens of thousands of families across the United States. Funded primarily by state budgets from federal funding for welfare reform and the cigarette settlement largesse in the 1990s, HFA is arguably the most recognized direct service prevention program promoted by PCA America.

Early expectations of program success led many funders, administrators, and evaluators to study only distal outcomes, such as the rate of official child maltreatment, bypassing the critical step of examining implementation closely, a common problem in social science (Durlak, 1997). Our focus on the implementation experiences suggests the following five lessons for benefiting from the HFA experiment and moving forward:

1. HFA is best considered as an organic, learning laboratory. Not only is HFA learning new ways to respond to the needs of its families, such as sustaining their interest in providing the best environment and learning experiences for children, but it is also learning more about the conditions that stymie protective interventions. HFA provides a needed real time laboratory of social and health interventions to better determine the effectiveness of home visitation and its delivery system, content, and quality. HFA offers comparisons of roles played by staffing structures, training and technical assistance, and supervision modalities; it provides an opportunity to understand more about the effect of certification and quality assurance. HFA's singular strength–its adaptability to the varied terrains of populations and neighborhoods–allows HFA to compare outcomes across differences and similarities of childrearing experiences. Similar to other public health initiatives with feedback loops for program improvement and quality assurance, HFA's dissemination of evaluations and research using the credentialing process make it a fluid work-in-progress (Oshana, Harding, Friedman, & Holton, 2005). HFA researchers can study how local adaptations, such as differences in community, host agency, and service provider characteristics; target population (risk factors); and services provided (based on community capacities) influence outcomes.

2. To learn from our experiences requires ongoing documentation in myriad formats–some likely to be more expensive than others but all necessary (Korbin & Coulton, 1997): randomized trials (Rosen, Manor, Engelhard, & Zucker, 2006), ethnographic interviews (Stack & Burton, 1994), and community surveys (Giachello et al., 2003). More consistent outcomes can be achieved in HFA once the empirical, albeit complex, question of model flexibility is addressed. One source of variation that is likely to persist–the average risk level of families served by a given program (Harding et al., 2004)–must be routinely assessed in ways that permit cross-site comparison and

testing of differences relative to outcomes. In addition, the original rationale for creating a flexible model, namely, the uniqueness of each community surrounding HFA sites, should be a central focus in process and outcome evaluation to understand how contextual factors impact program effectiveness. Currently, an understanding of the risks to children and caregivers from their neighborhood context is an underdeveloped attribute of both HFA and PCA America (Meyer, Armstrong-Cohen, & Batista, 2005; Sidelinger et al., 2005).

3. As currently implemented, good outcome data from one site cannot be generalized to another program site, even in the same state; conversely, bad outcomes can be explained away as site-specific. More sophisticated methods are needed to examine how family, provider, site, and community factors interact and combine to mediate implementation indicators. For instance, the City of Hampton (VA) has shown community-wide impacts following the implementation of HFA (Galano & Huntington, 2002). Although most evaluative attention is focused on HFA's direct services to individual children and families, its ecological underpinnings and its systems approach to implementation have lead to community-wide change. Much remains to be learned and applied when an additional critical element, for example, the therapeutic expectation of parental partnerships in the implementation of home visiting services, is added to the model and implemented at the local level (Carnahan, Nelson, & Gordon, 1999). Identifying and utilizing outside sources of evaluation that promote timely feedback to both participants and practitioners is fundamental.

4. As Gomby et al. (1999) suggested, the culprit for poor outcomes with HFA could be found in program implementation. Although HFA has taken steps to ensure its fidelity by establishing a credentialing process, empirical evidence from credentialed vs. non-credentialed sites remains to be evaluated to ascertain whether fidelity to the model *as implemented* translates into greater benefits to families. Additionally, building the capacity to answer questions measuring stakeholder commitments to HFA, short-term "customer" satisfaction with the program and long-term impact on families, and a commitment to implement long-term evaluative outcomes will be necessary.

5. Although ecologic theory is oriented to examine multi-level causality, the prevention focus of HFA has been aimed at one level–enhancing parental skills. HFA predominantly reaches those families who

possess the greatest risks and the fewest resources for change. As implemented, local HFA sites deemphasize distal influences (outside the family), thereby limiting prevention opportunities from other environmental contributors (Belsky, 1980; Garbarino & Kostelny, 1994). In implementing HFA, acknowledging and addressing larger contextual influences such as poverty or "concentrated disadvantage" with home visitation services would suggest a readiness to combat poverty as the comprehensive community initiatives of the 1980s and '90s had done (Auspos & Kubisch, 2004). HFA has yet to design, for example, a community engagement practice to counteract concentrated disadvantage and its community accomplices, namely violence on the street and in the home.

HFA began as a program to help parents and caregivers support their children's growth and development. Acknowledging that more needs to be done to improve the HFA model–strengthening its operational infrastructure, training, and evaluation–is not a signal of its demise. On the contrary, direct service programs that support every child's right to grow into adulthood without the trauma of abuse and neglect are needed. Child abuse prevention occurs when deleterious behaviors are diverted, changed, or transformed. Finding the best means to accomplish prevention requires help from all quarters beginning with caregivers and their families. The latter, as repositories of their children's hopes, generally seek and respond to overtures of support and assistance. How parents are helped by their communities and the society at-large underscores or undermines the future of all children.

NOTES

1. Now referred to as the *Nurse Family Partnership Program* (Olds, Eckenrode, Henderson, Kitzman, Powers, Cole et al., 1997; Olds et al., 2004).

2. For another example of externalizing events impacting childrearing see Molnar et al. (2003, 2005) studies on violence outside the home and its links to physical aggressiveness toward children.

3. This article did not examine family outcomes in relation to implementation of HFA; to summarize the research evidence concerning HFA family outcomes is a complex task taken up elsewhere in this volume (see Harding, Galano, Martin, Huntington & Schellenbach, this issue).

REFERENCES

Aspen Institute Roundtable on Community Change (2004). *Structural racism and community building*. Washington, DC: Aspen Institute.

Auspos, P., & Kubisch, A. C. (2004). *Building knowledge about community change: Moving beyond evaluation*. New York: Aspen Institute.

Azar, S. T., Povilaitis, T. Y., Lauretti, A. F., & Pouquette, C. L. (1998). The current status of etiological theories in intrafamilial child maltreatment. In J. R. Lutzker (Ed.), *Handbook of child abuse research and treatment*. New York: Plenum Press.

Bandura, A. (1971). *Social learning theory*. New York: General Learning Press.

Belsky, J. (1980). Child maltreatment: An ecological integration. *American Psychologist*, *35*(4), 320-335.

Black, T., Powell, J. L., Clay, M., & McDill, P. (2000). Healthy Families Connecticut: Final outcome evaluation report of a home visitation program to enhance positive parenting and reduce child maltreatment. Center for Social Research, University of Hartford, West Hartford, CT.

Bowlby, J. (1988). *A secure base: Parent-child attachment and healthy human development*. New York: Basic Books.

Bowlby, J., Ainsworth, M., Boston, M., & Rosenbluth, D. (1956). The effects of mother-child separation: A follow-up study. *British Journal of Medical Psychology*, *29*(2), 11-247.

Brooks-Gunn, J. (1995). Children in families in communities: Risk and prevention in the Bronfenbrenner tradition. In P. Moen, G. H. Elder Jr., & K. Luscher (Eds.), *Examining lives in context: Perspectives on the ecology of human development* (pp. 467-519). Washington, DC: American Psychological Association.

Bronfenbrenner, U. (1977). Toward an experimental ecology of human development. *American Psychologist*, *32*, 513-531.

Brooks-Gunn, J., Duncan, G. J., & Aber, J. L. (1997). *Neighborhood poverty: Context and consequences for children* (Vol. 1). New York: Russell Sage Foundation.

Carnahan, S., Nelson, C. E., & Gordon, T. R. (1999). A community-based approach to preventing child maltreatment. In R. N. Roberts & P. R. Magrab (Eds.), *Where children live: Solutions for serving young children and their families. Advances in Applied Developmental Psychology* (Vol. 17). Stamford, CT: Ablex Publishing.

Centers for Disease Control and Prevention (2003). First reports evaluating the effectiveness of strategies for preventing violence: Early childhood home visitation and firearms laws. Findings from the Task Force on Community Preventive Services. *Morbidity and Mortality Weekly Report*, *52* (No. RR-14), 1-9.

Chaffin, M. (2005). Letter to the editor. *Child Abuse and Neglect*, *29*, 241-249.

Chaffin, M. (2004). Is it time to rethink healthy start/healthy families? *Child Abuse and Neglect*, *28*, 589-595.

Chaffin, M., & Friedrich, B. (2004). Evidence-based treatments in child abuse and neglect. *Children and Youth Services Review*, *26*, 1097-1113.

Cicchetti, D., & Lynch, M. (1993). Toward an ecological/transactional model of community violence and child maltreatment: Consequences for children's development. In D. Reiss, J. E. Richters, M. Radke-Yarrow, & D. Scharff (Eds.), *Children and violence* (pp. 96-118). New York: Guilford Press.

Coulton, C. J., Korbin, J. E., Su, M., & Chow, J. (1995). Community level factors and child maltreatment rates. *Child Development, 66*, 1262-1276.

Daro, D. (1998). *Public opinion and behaviors regarding child abuse prevention: 1998 Survey. Working paper number 804.* Chicago: Prevent Child Abuse America.

Daro, D. (1999). *Public opinion and behaviors regarding child abuse prevention: 1999 Survey. Working paper number 840.* Chicago: Prevent Child Abuse America.

Daro, D., & Donnelly, A. C. (2003). Charting the waves of prevention: Two steps forward, one step back. *Child Abuse and Neglect, 26*, 731-742.

Daro, D., Jones, E., & McCurdy, K. (1993). *Preventing child abuse: An evaluation of services to high-risk families.* Chicago: National Committee to Prevent Child Abuse.

Daro, D., McCurdy, K., & Harding, K. (1998). *The role of home visiting in preventing child abuse: An evaluation of the Hawaii Healthy Start program.* Chicago: National Committee to Prevent Child Abuse.

Derezotes, D., Poertner, J., & Testa, M. (2005). *Race matters in child welfare: The overrepresentation of African American children in the system.* (Eds.) Washington, DC: CWLA Press.

Diaz, J., Oshana, D., & Harding, K. (2004). *Healthy Families America: 2003 annual profile of program sites.* Chicago: Prevent Child Abuse America.

Donnelly, A. C. (1983). *An approach to preventing child abuse* (2nd ed.). Chicago: Prevent Child Abuse America.

Duggan, A., McFarlane, E., Fuddy, L., Burrell, L., Higman, S. M., Windham, A. et al. (2004). Randomized trial of a statewide program of home visiting to prevent child abuse: Impact in preventing child abuse and neglect. *Child Abuse and Neglect, 28*, 597-622.

Durlak, J. A. (1997). *Successful prevention programs for children and adolescents.* New York: Plenum Press.

Eckenrode, J., Ganzel, B., Henderson, C. R., Smith, E., Olds, D., Powers, J. et al. (2000). Preventing child abuse and neglect with a program of nurse home visitation: The limiting effects of domestic violence. *Journal of the American Medical Association, 284*, 1385-1391.

Egeland, B., Sroufe, L. A., & Erikson, M. F. (1983). The developmental consequences of different patterns of maltreatment. *Child Abuse and Neglect, 7*, 459-169.

Felitti, V. J., Anda, R. F., Nordenberg, D., Williamson, D. F., Spitz, A. M., Edwards, V. et al. (1998). Relationship of childhood abuse and household dysfunction to many of the leading causes of death in adults: The adverse childhood experiences (ACE) study. *American Journal of Preventive Medicine, 14*, 245-258.

Galano, J., & Huntington, L. (2002). *FY 2002 Healthy Families Partnership Benchmark Study: Measuring Community-Wide Impact.* Prepared by the Applied Social Psychology Research Institute, College of William and Mary, Williamsburg, VA.

Garbarino, J., & Barry, F. (1997). The community context of child abuse and neglect. In J. Garbarino & J. Eckenrode (Eds.), *Understanding abusive families: An ecological approach to theory and practice* (pp. 56-85). San Francisco: Jossey-Bass.

Garbarino, J., & Kostelny, K. (1994). Child maltreatment as a community problem. *Child Abuse and Neglect, 16*, 455-464.

Giachello, A., Arrom, J., Davis, M., Sayad., J., Ramirez, D., Nandi, C. et al. (2003). Reducing diabetes health disparities through community-based participatory action research: The Chicago southeast diabetes community action coalition. *Public Health Reports, 118*, 309-323.

Golden, R. (1992). *Disposable children: America's child welfare system.* Belmont, CA: Wadsworth Publishing Co.

Gomby, D., Culross, P., & Behrman, R. (1999). Home visiting: Recent program evaluations–Analysis and recommendations. *The Future of Children, 9*(1), 4-26.

Green, L. W., & Kreuter, M. W. (2004). *Health program planning: An educational and ecological approach.* Columbus, OH: McGraw-Hill.

Guterman, N. (1999). Enrollment strategies in early home visitation to prevent physical child abuse and neglect and the "universal versus targeted" debate: A meta-analysis of population-based and screening-based programs. *Child Abuse and Neglect, 23*, 863-890.

Guterman, N. (2001). *Stopping child maltreatment before it starts: Emerging horizons in early home visitation services.* Thousand Oaks, CA: Sage.

Halpern, R. (1995). *Rebuilding the inner city: A history of neighborhood initiatives to address poverty in the United States.* New York: Columbia University Press.

Hammond, W. R. (2003). Public health and child maltreatment prevention: The role of the Centers for Disease Control and Prevention. *Child Maltreatment, 8*, 81-83.

Harding, K., Galano, J., Martin, J., Huntington, L., & Schellenbach, C. (in press). Healthy Families America effectiveness: A comprehensive review of outcomes.

Harding, K. A. (2002). Child abuse prevention efforts: Strengthening families, protecting children. In A. Giardino & E. Giardino (Eds.), *Recognition of child abuse for the mandated reporter.* St. Louis, MO: G. W. Medical Publishing.

Harding, K., Friedman, L., & Diaz J. (2003). *Healthy Families America: 2001 annual profile of program sites.* Chicago: Prevent Child Abuse America.

Harding, K. A., Reid, R., Oshana, D., Holton, J., & Representatives of the Healthy Families America Research Practice Council (2004). Initial results of the national Healthy Families America implementation study: A report submitted to the David and Lucille Packard Foundation. Chicago: Prevent Child Abuse America.

Harrington, D., & Dubowitz, H. (1999). Preventing child maltreatment. In R. L. Hampton (Ed.), *Family violence: Prevention and treatment* (2nd ed.). Thousand Oaks, CA: Sage.

Harway, M. (2000). Families experiencing violence. In W. Nichols & M. Pace-Nichols (Eds.), *Handbook of family development and intervention.* New York: John Wiley & Sons.

Harway, M., & Hansen, M. (1993). Therapist perceptions of family violence. In M. Hansen & M. Harway (Eds.), *Battering and family therapy: A feminist perspective.* Thousand Oaks, CA: Sage Publications.

Healthy Families Credentialing Manual (1999). Chicago: Prevent Child Abuse America.

Johnson, S., & Lebow, J. (2000). The "coming of age" of family therapy: A decade review. *Journal of Marital & Family Therapy, 26*, 23-38.

Kempe, C. H. (1976a). Approaches to preventing child abuse:The health visitors concept. *American Journal of Diseases of Children, 130*, 941-947.

Kempe, C. H. (1976b). Predicting and preventing child abuse: Establishing children's rights by assuring access to health care through the health visitors concept. In *Proceedings of the First National Conference on Child Abuse and Neglect, January*

4-7, 1976 (pp. 67-75). Washington, DC: US Department of Health, Education and Welfare.

Kempe, C. H., Silverman, F. N., Steele, B., Droegemueller, W., & Silver, H. R. (1962). The battered child syndrome. *Journal of the American Medical Association, 181,* 17-24.

Kempe, R. S., & Kempe, C. H. (1976). Child abuse. In J. Bruner, M. Cole, & B. Lloyd (Eds.), *The developing child series.* Cambridge, MA: Harvard University Press.

Kessler, S. R. (2004). The impact of fidelity on program quality in the Healthy Families America programs. Unpublished master's thesis. University of South Florida.

Korbin, J., & Coulton, C. (1997). Understanding the neighborhood context for children and families: Combining epidemiological and ethnographic approaches. In J. Brooks-Gunn, G. J. Duncan, & J. L. Aber (Eds.), *Neighborhood poverty* (Vol. 2, pp. 65-79). New York: Sage.

Korfmacher, J. (2000). The Kempe family stress inventory: A review. *Child Abuse and Neglect, 24,* 129-140.

Kubisch, A., Auspos, P., Brown, P., Chaskin, R., Fulbright-Anderson, K., & Hamilton R. (2002). *Voices from the field II: Reflections on comprehensive community change.* Washington, DC: Aspen Institute.

Landsverk, J., Carillio, T., Connelly, C. D., Ganger, W. C., Slymen, D. J., Newton, R. R. et al. (2002). *Healthy Families San Diego clinical trial: Technical report.* San Diego Children's Hospital and Health Center, Child and Adolescent Services Research Center.

Lane, W. G., Rubin, D. M., Monteith, R., & Christian, C. W. (2002). Racial differences in the evaluation of pediatric fractures for physical abuse. *Journal of the American Medical Association, 288,* 1603-1609.

Leventhal, J. M. (2004). Getting prevention right: Maintaining the status quo is not an option. *Child Abuse and Neglect, 29,* 209-213.

Maas, H. S. (1975). Children's environments and child welfare. In W. C. Sze (Ed.), *Human life cycle* (pp. 193-206). New York: Jason Aronson, Inc.

Macdonald, G. (2001). *Effective interventions for child abuse and neglect: An evidence based approach to planning and evaluating interventions.* Chichester, UK: John Wiley.

Marable, M. (2001). Racism and sexism. In Paula S. Rothenberg, (Ed.), *Race, class, and gender in the United States* (5th ed.). New York: Worth Publishers.

Mendoza, J., Katz, L., Robertson, A., & Rothenberg, D. (2003). *Connecting with parents in the early years.* Champaign, IL: U.S. Department of Education.

Meyer, D., Armstrong-Cohen, A., & Batista, M. (2005). How a community-based organization and an academic health center are creating an effective partnership for training and service. *Academic Medicine, 80*(4), 1-7.

Molnar, B. E. (2004). Neighborhood predictors of concealed firearm carrying among children and adolescents. *Pediatric Adolescent Medicine, 158,* 657-664.

Molnar, B. E. (2005). Violent behavior by girls report violent victimization. *Arch. Pediatric Adolescent Medicine, 159,* 731-739.

Molnar, B. E., Buka, S. L., Brennan, R. T., Holton, J. K., & Earls, F. (2003). A multilevel study of neighborhoods and parent-to-child physical aggression: Results from the project on human development in Chicago neighborhoods. *Child Maltreatment, 8*(2), 84-97.

National Research Council (1993). *Understanding child abuse and neglect*. Washington, DC: National Academy Press.

Nelson, B. (1984). *Making an issue of child abuse*. Chicago: University of Chicago Press.

Oates, K. (1982). Child abuse: A community concern. In K. Oates (Ed.), *Child abuse: A community concern* (pp. 1-12). New York: Brunner/Mazel.

Olds, D. L., Henderson, C. R., Chamberlin, R., & Tatelbaum, R. (1986). Preventing child abuse and neglect: A randomized trial of nurse home visitation. *Pediatrics, 78*(1), 65-78.

Olds, D., Eckenrode, J., Henderson, C., Kitzman, H., Powers, J., Cole, R. et al. (1997). Long-term effects of home visitation on maternal life course and child abuse and neglect: Fifteen-year follow-up of a randomized trial. *Journal of the American Medical Association, 278*, 637-643.

Olds, D. L., Robinson, J., O'Brien, R., Luckey, D. W., Pettitt, L. M., Henderson, C. R. et al. (2004). Home visiting by paraprofessionals and by nurses: A randomized, controlled trial. *Pediatrics, 110*, 486-496.

Orkow, B. (1985). Implementation of a family stress checklist. *Child Abuse and Neglect, 9*, 405-410.

Oshana, D., Harding, K., Friedman, L., & Holton, J. (2005). Letter to the Editor. *Child Abuse and Neglect, 29*, 219-228.

Partnership guide for Healthy Families America (HFA) sites and children's hospitals committed to supporting new parents (1998). Alexandria, VA: National Association of Children's Hospitals and Related Institutions.

Roberts, D. (2002). *Shattered bonds: The color of child welfare*. New York: Basic Civitas Books.

Rosen, L., Manor, O., Engelhard, D., & Zucker, D. (2006). In defense of the randomized controlled trial for health promotion research. *American Journal of Public Health, 96*, 1181-1186.

Sampson, R. J. (1997). Collective regulation of adolescent misbehavior: Validation results from eighty Chicago neighborhoods. *Journal of Adolescent Research, 12*, 227-244.

Sampson, R. J., Raudenbush, S., & Earls, F. (1997). Neighborhoods and violent crime: A multilevel study of collective efficacy. *Science, 27*, 918-924.

Schumaker, J., Smith Slep, A., & Heyman, R. E. (2001). Risk factors for child neglect. *Aggression and Violent Behavior, 6*, 231-254.

Sherwood, K. E. (2005). Evaluating home visitation: A case study of evaluation at the David and Lucile Packard Foundation. *New Directions for Evaluation, 105*, 59-78.

Sidelinger, D., Meyer, D., Blaschke, G., Hametz, P., Batista, M., Salguero, R. et al. (2005). Communities as teachers: Learning to deliver culturally effective care in pediatrics. *Pediatrics, 115*, 1160-1164.

Stack, C., & Burton, L. (1994). Kinscripts: Reflections of family, generation, and culture. In E. N. Glenn, G. Chang, & L. R. Forcey (Eds.), *Mothering: Ideology, experience, and agency* (pp. 33-44) New York: Routledge.

Trickett, P., & Shellenbach, C. J. (Eds.) (1998). *Violence against children in the family and the community*. Washington, DC: American Psychological Association.

US Department of Health and Human Services (DHHS), US Advisory Board on Child Abuse and Neglect (1990). *Child abuse and neglect: Critical first steps in response to a national emergency*. Washington, DC: US Government Printing Office.

US Department of Health and Human Services (DHHS), US Advisory Board on Child Abuse and Neglect (1991). *Creating caring communities: Blueprint for an effective federal policy on child abuse and neglect* (Rep. No. 9-1991). Washington, DC: US Government Printing Office.

US Department of Health and Human Services (DHHS), National Center on Child Abuse and Neglect. (1996). *The third national incidence study of child abuse and neglect.* Washington, DC: US Government Printing Office.

US Department of Health and Human Services (2000). *Healthy people 2010* (2nd ed., Vols. 1-2). Washington, DC: US Government Printing Office.

Wasik, B. H., & Bryant, D. M. (2001). *Home visitation: Procedures for helping families* (2nd ed.) Thousand Oakes: Sage.

doi:10.1300/J005v34n01_02

APPENDIX 1. A Short History of Hawaii Family Stress Center[1]

1975: Gail Breakey and Barbara Naki of the Hawaii Family Stress Center visited the E. Henry Kempe Center in Denver, CO for training in establishing child abuse programs in Hawaii, funded by an early NCCAN grant. They met with Dr. Kempe, who had developed a home visiting program using paraprofessionals to prevent child abuse and a scale to differentiate between families who would or would not need such a program.

1975: The first Hawaii home visiting programs started in at Kapiolani Medical Center in Honolulu, utilizing the Kempe scale and providing short term, approximately 18 months, home visiting services for families referred by the hospital or community providers. This program was quickly replicated on the neighbor islands with one small program on each island, i.e., 1-2 home visitors with a half-time time coordinator who also conducted the Kempe scale. The goal was to prevent child abuse.

1984: Hawaii Family Support Center, seeing promising results of the early program, recognized that to maximize impact, a pilot program would be needed to establish that could lead to implementation of a statewide system. The strategy of the pilot project would be to serve all families with a newborn within a specific geographic area and to demonstrate the potential for large scale prevention of child abuse. The program would serve infants from birth to age five with a primary goal of preventing child abuse and a secondary focus on improving child development. The Kempe Family Stress Checklist was used to determine those families who might benefit from home visiting services, and to offer community resource linkage to all other families. Legislative advocacy resulted in funding for this program starting in 1985; successful outcomes enabled incremental expansion across the state.

In 1989, an article appeared in the *New York Times* about the Healthy Start program and the value of home visiting as an effective vehicle to prevent child abuse and neglect. The article featured the Hawaii Healthy Start program as a premier strategy to prevent child abuse and neglect. The Associated Press picked up the article and newspapers across the country published the story. Individuals from many states contacted the Hawaii Family Support Center, including Arizona, Virginia, and New Mexico where advocates hoped to implement similar programs.

1991: Betsy Dew and Gail Breakey presented on Hawaii Healthy Start at the National Center on Child Abuse & Neglect Conference in Denver. Dr. Richard Krugman, successor to Dr. Kempe at the Denver Center and chair of the U.S. Advisory Board on Child Abuse & Neglect, held a press conference on the findings of the 1991 Advisory Boards national report on child abuse. He recommended home visitation as a viable strategy to prevent child abuse and neglect; he described the Hawaii Healthy Start program as the "star" of home visiting programs. Ann Cohn-Donnelly and January Scott of National Committee to Prevent Child Abuse (now Prevent Child Abuse America or PCA America) met with Dew and Breakey to discuss options for a potential proposal to Ronald McDonald's Children's Charities. It was agreed that a combination of state and regional meetings to provide information on home visiting as a strategy to prevent child abuse, and provision of training and technical assistance to organizations interested in starting programs would be the approach taken for this grant, with the intent of launching a national home visiting initiative.

[1] Contributed by Kate Whitaker, Arizona HFA Director. Used with permission.

APPENDIX 2. The Healthy Families America Critical Elements

1. Initiate services prenatally or at birth.

2. Use a standardized (i.e., consistent for all families) assessment tool to systematically identify families who are most in need of services.

3. Offer services voluntarily and use positive, persistent outreach efforts to build family trust.

4. Offer services intensively (i.e., at least once a week) with well-defined criteria for increasing or decreasing intensity of service and over the long term (i.e., three to five years).

5. Services should be culturally competent such that the staff understands, acknowledges, and respects cultural differences among participants; and materials used should reflect the cultural, linguistic, geographic, racial, and ethnic diversity of the population served.

6. Services should focus on supporting the parent(s) as well as supporting parent-child interaction and child development.

7. At a minimum, all families should be linked to a medical provider to assure optimal health and development (e.g., timely immunizations, well-child care, etc.) Depending on the family's needs, they may also be linked to additional services such as financial, food, and housing assistance programs, school readiness programs, child care, job training programs, family support centers, substance abuse treatment programs, and domestic violence shelters.

8. Services should be provided by staff with limited caseloads to assure that home visitors have an adequate amount of time to spend with each family to meet their unique and varying needs and to plan for future activities (i.e., for most communities no more than 15 families per home visitor on the most intense service level).

9. Service providers should be selected because of their personal characteristics (i.e., nonjudgmental, compassionate, able to establish a trusting relationship, etc.), their willingness to work in or their experience working with culturally diverse communities, and their skills to do the job.

10. Service providers should have a framework, based on education or experience, for handling the variety of experiences they may encounter when working with at-risk families.

11. Service providers should receive intensive training specific to their role to understand the essential components of family assessment and home visitation.

12. Service providers should receive ongoing, effective supervision so that they are able to develop realistic and effective plans to empower families to meet their objectives; to understand why a family may not be making progress and how to work with the family more effectively; and to express their concerns and frustrations.

APPENDIX 3: Examples of Credentialing Questions

---

1. Initiate services prenatally or at birth.

1-1. Program ensures it identifies **participants** in the **target population** for services either while mother is pregnant (prenatally) and/or at the birth of baby.

1-1.A. The program has a description of the **target population** that includes key demographic information such as number of resident live births per year, number of women of child-bearing age, number of single parents, age of the **target population**, and race/ethnicity/linguistic/**cultural characteristics** of population and places where the population is found (e.g., local hospitals, prenatal clinics, high schools, etc.).

EVIDENCE 1-1.A.

Pre-site: Please submit a description of the program's **target population** (including **demographic characteristics** described in standard 1-1.A.).

On-site: Interview staff assigned to maintain information on **target population**.

1-1.A. RATING INDICATORS

3 - The program has a description of the **target population** and identifies organizations within the community in which the **target population** can be found. Both the description and identification are comprehensive and up-to-date.

2 - The program has a description of the **target population** and identifies organizations within the community in which the **target population** can be found. The community services and supports while sufficient for its needs, could be more comprehensive.

1 - Any of the following: program does not have a description of the **target population**; program does not identify organizations within the community in which the **target population** can be found; and/or the description and/or identification have major information gaps.

Source: Healthy Families Credentialing Manual, 2004. Used with permission.

Healthy Families America®
Research Practice Network:
A Unique Partnership
to Integrate Prevention Science and Practice

Joseph Galano

College of William & Mary

Cynthia J. Schellenbach

Oakland University

SUMMARY. The goal of the Healthy Families America Research to Practice Network (RPN) was to foster communication among academic researchers, community-based evaluators, and practitioners to integrate science-based prevention practices into practice settings. The RPN goals were guided by and are a response to the limitations of past and current research paradigms in the social sciences. Accomplishments included creation of a 40-member researcher-practitioner council, development of a national Program Information Management System, and completion of a 4-year national Implementation Study, employing data from over 100 sites in nine states. The discussion examines what was learned about this rare experiment in creating practitioner-scientist partnerships and

Address correspondence to: Joseph Galano, Department of Psychology, College of William and Mary, P.O. Box 8795, Williamsburg, VA 23187-8795 (E-mail: jxgala@wm.edu).

[Haworth co-indexing entry note]: "Healthy Families America® Research Practice Network: A Unique Partnership to Integrate Prevention Science and Practice." Galano, Joseph, and Cynthia J. Schellenbach. Co-published simultaneously in *Journal of Prevention & Intervention in the Community* (The Haworth Press, Inc.) Vol. 34, No. 1/2, 2007, pp. 39-66; and: *The Healthy Families America® Initiative: Integrating Research, Theory and Practice* (ed: Joseph Galano) The Haworth Press, 2007, pp. 39-66. Single or multiple copies of this article are available for a fee from The Haworth Document Delivery Service [1-800-HAWORTH, 9:00 a.m. - 5:00 p.m. (EST). E-mail address: docdelivery@haworthpress.com].

doi:10.1300/J005v34n01_03

the impact of the RPN on child abuse and neglect prevention. A five-year plan to sustain and strengthen a practice-research collaborative is recommended. doi:10.1300/J005v34n01_03 *[Article copies available for a fee from The Haworth Document Delivery Service: 1-800-HAWORTH. E-mail address: <docdelivery@haworthpress.com> Website: <http://www.HaworthPress.com> © 2007 by The Haworth Press, Inc. All rights reserved.]*

KEYWORDS. Research to practice, researcher-practitioner, prevention, community intervention, partnership networks

INTRODUCTION

More research is required to integrate prevention science and practice. In fact, funded scientific investigations on effective ways to foster the integration of science-based prevention and field-based practice have been rare. The Healthy Families America (HFA) Research Practice Network (RPN) represents a unique partnership of researchers and practitioners with support from Prevent Child Abuse America (PCA America) and the Carnegie Foundation. The Network was originally created to bridge the gap between academic researchers and community-based researchers of home visitation programs. Specifically, the RPN was described as a unique experiment (Kahn, 1993) because it represented one of the few field-driven research collaboratives in the country. The goals of the initiative were to: (a) improve the quantity and quality of HFA evaluations and programs; (b) create a common database for describing HFA programs, participants, and outcomes; (c) encourage secondary analyses of existing evaluative data on home visitation; and (d) identify critical research questions and the most effective way to address these questions. The purpose of this article is to chronicle the history and accomplishments of the network in relation to these goals. The article presents a framework that is useful to the RPN for illustrating the various barriers between prevention science and practice and the bridges to overcome them. It discusses the goals of the RPN, offers a detailed plan for sustaining and growing the collaborative, and posits the need for national leadership and funding.

Research on the developmental impact of child abuse has proliferated over the past 40 years (Kendall-Tackett, Williams, & Finkelhor, 1993; Tricket & McBride-Chang, 1995; Widom, 1989). Such research has moved the field forward by defining the types of maltreatment (Cicchetti &

Lynch, 1993; Kempe et al., 1962) and the impact of abuse on the developmental process. National research has documented the incidence and severity of abuse in the United States (National Incidence Study, NCCAN, 1996; American Association for Protecting Children, 1988). On the basis of this research, there have been calls for Congress to study the problem (U.S. Advisory Board on Child Abuse and Neglect, 1990) and appropriate funds for research and services. As a result of these efforts, half of the American public believes that child abuse and neglect are among the most serious public health issues confronting the United States, outranking substance abuse (Daro, 2000). According to the National Advisory Board on Child Abuse and Neglect (1993), child abuse is a serious social problem, and the prevention of child abuse is cited as a targeted objective for the nation in *Healthy People 2010* (U.S. Department of Health and Human Services [USDHHS], 2000).

Despite strides in understanding, treating, and preventing child abuse and neglect, it remains one of the most significant public health problems in the United States. In 2000, nearly 2 million reports involving 2.7 million children were referred for investigation (USDHHS, 2003). Of these children, approximately 879,000 were found to be victims of maltreatment. The impact on our nation is profound. Survivors inherit a deplorable long-term legacy that includes mental retardation, intellectual and social deficiencies, major adult health problems, and increased risks for school failure, delinquency, and violent behavior (Cicchetti & Toth, 2000; National Research Council and Institute of Medicine, 2000).

In recognition of the seriousness of this problem, a great deal of research aimed at increasing our understanding of the etiology and prevention of child abuse and neglect has been undertaken. Considerable federal and state funding supported the development and testing of specific prevention activities (parent education programs, skill-based curricula for children, respite programs, and family resources centers) as well as large-scale community-based programs, such as Nurse Family Partnership, HFA, Home Instruction Program for Parents of Pre-school Youngsters, and Parents as Teachers (Baker, Piotrkowski, & Brooks-Gunn, 1999; Olds et al., 1999).

After extensive review of the child abuse and neglect literature by a number of governmental and private organizations, home visitation was identified as "the most promising strategy for developing or improving access to early intervention services that can help at-risk families become healthier and more self-sufficient" (Government Accounting Office, 1990). The U.S. Advisory Board on Child Abuse and Neglect urged the federal government to begin planning for the implementation of a universal,

voluntary, neonatal home visitation system. In response to the recommendation, the National Committee to Prevent Child Abuse, in partnership
with Ronald McDonald Children's Charities, launched HFA in February
1992. As of June 1996, HFA programs were operating in almost 200 communities in 35 states, and today HFA operates in over 430 communities in
about 40 states.

Although HFA's leaders believed that increased dissemination of the
model was the correct course of action, the scientific knowledge available
to guide the national initiative was incomplete. Importantly, there was
very little systematic exchange of information among researchers. At the
various sites, evaluators, both those with the resources to conduct randomized trials and those conducting a wide array of non-experimental
evaluations, had limited opportunities to exchange information or build
on each other's efforts (Daro & Harding, 1999).

From the beginning, PCA America recognized the needs for research
on the etiology, treatment, and prevention of child maltreatment. In 1986,
PCA America created its National Center on Child Abuse Prevention Research (National Center) with a mission to bridge the gap between
researchers and practitioners. To date, the National Center is at the fore-
front of surveillance and evaluation of child maltreatment prevention
efforts.

The National Center was based on the developmental ecological approach to child maltreatment (Belsky, 1980; Garbarino & Barry, 1997).
Most models of child maltreatment recognize that factors in the child, the
family, the community, and the society contribute to child maltreatment.
Amelioration of this problem requires recognition of the multiple causality
of child maltreatment, multiple-component intervention, and prevention
programs that reach children, families, organizations, and communities
(Daro, 1996). Current research on child abuse prevention underscores
that these efforts should be evidence-based, actionable, and practical
(Green, 2002). However, there are gaps between research and practice
that severely limit the dissemination of evidence-based child abuse prevention strategies, research efforts, and policy (Daro & Cohn-Donnelly,
2002; Tricket & Pizzagotti, 1999). Moreover, there exist serious problems in
community participation, interpretation, and application of research findings (Maton, Schellenbach, Leadbeater, & Solarz, 1999). These complex
issues are not unique to child abuse prevention, but mirror the challenges
faced in the prevention of substance abuse, violence, and mental illness
(Green, 2001; Patton, 2002).

PCA America conceptualizes child maltreatment and its prevention as
a public health challenge rather than an individualistic problem involving
only law enforcement, child welfare, medical personnel, and the accused

parents. PCA America was one of the first organizations to encourage states and localities, through its nationwide system of chapters, to become involved in implementing child abuse and neglect prevention programs on the local and national levels. This recognition of the importance of ecology has lead to a community development approach that attempts to mobilize many sectors of the community, including human service agencies, to develop public health solutions to public health problems. Over the past decade, the strategy of implementing community-level interventions combining multiple strategies across multiple settings has been embraced as a promising approach for preventing substance abuse, delinquency, and violence (Wandersman & Florin, 2003).

The promise of mobilizing the community in prevention efforts, however, is often not realized when communities are left on their own to discover and utilize findings from emerging prevention science. Allowing local initiatives to make painstakingly little progress has been a wasteful process and will hinder future growth of community-based prevention initiatives. Most wasteful of all has been the absence of well-funded, concerted attempts to learn systematically from current experience and to disseminate that learning to those responsible for community-change initiatives, to those who make relevant policy in the private and public sector, and to the general public (Schorr, 1997). Indeed, recent research has identified barriers that limit the integration of research, practice, and policy. The barriers include organizational factors, differences in theoretical orientations, cultural differences, and lack of readiness in the community. All of these issues function as disincentives for the collaboration needed to advance the field (Lamb, Greenlick, & McCarty, 1998). The promise of prevention will never be realized without appropriate infrastructures to link research, practice, and policy. PCA America has established a goal of creating an infrastructure that strives to integrate research, practice, and policy. Thus, with the support of the Robert Wood Johnson Foundation, PCA America created the HFA Research Network in 1996.

COMPONENTS OF THE EARLY DEVELOPMENT OF THE HFA RESEARCH NETWORK

Throughout the United States, research programs funded by federal agencies and foundations are attempting to build a prevention science which delineates what works, for what populations, and for what types of problems (Morrissey et al., 1997). To be effective, however, prevention science must be transformed into prevention practice. Programs aimed at the major public health problems in our country such as substance abuse, child abuse, youth violence, AIDS, and adolescent pregnancy reach millions of people in America each day. Most of those programs, similar to HFA, consist of both research and community-driven prevention. The authors underscore that the categories of research are a typology rather than a dichotomy, and integration of the components is likely to be very effective in the field (Wandersman & Florin, 2003).

Research-driven prevention is directed by academics or university-based researchers. Often these efforts consist of randomized experimental designs and a series of clinical trials. These trials are costly, are typically funded by federal agencies, and are few in number. Two advantages of the research-driven prevention efforts are the strengths of the research methodology and the ability of the researcher to determine program impact by using a randomized control group design. Disadvantages are that the findings have limited impact at the community level, because pilot programs are usually too expensive to implement, are typically not sufficiently manualized for communities to easily adopt, and generally discourage sites from tailoring interventions to address local circumstances. Moreover, many health and human service sites do not allow experimental designs due to ethical issues and policy regulations.

In contrast to research-driven prevention, community-driven prevention originates within the community setting. One common mode of community prevention involves the use of community coalitions which mobilize individuals and organizations from various community sectors such as education, business, or religious settings with the goal of instigating community change. Change occurs through the processes of collaborative planning, implementation, and research evaluation. Ownership of the coalition, its change processes, and outcomes are community-driven in nature. The Hampton Healthy Families Partnership in Virginia and the Healthy Start Oakland partnership in Michigan are both examples of community coalitions that have documented positive outcomes for children and parents (Galano & Huntington, 2002).

There are many challenges to developing comprehensive community-based prevention programs that would account for the limited findings, in general, and in the child abuse and neglect arena specifically. These include the complexity of the problem, limited resources, staff and participant mobility, the lack of a mandate to cooperate, and modest community buy-in. Moreover, most community-based prevention programs have not consistently used the scientific information available regarding best practices and effective preventive interventions when designing and implementing community-based programs. Because of the lack of time and resources, programs seldom develop a well-delineated theory of action that will guide the development of goals, prevention services, and evaluation domains.

The challenges that HFA has confronted mirror the challenges that have confronted researchers in the field of prevention science: (a) building the knowledge base of prevention science, (b) exploring bridges and barriers between practice and science, and (c) developing effective prevention programs. Prevention scientists developed a framework (Morrissey et al., 1997) that integrates the current state of prevention practice, the contributions of prevention science, and the barriers that limit the transfer of knowledge between practice and science. These issues, depicted in Figure 1, have implications for the state of prevention practice and ways to improve it.

Figure 1 also depicts a gap between science and practice that is not unique to the field of prevention. Indeed, such a gap exists in virtually every field. Over the last 10 years, psychologists have paid increased attention to methods to bridge this gap. One prominent way is the technology transfer approach (Baker, David, & Soucy, 1995). This approach, delineated also in the Institute of Medicine (IOM) model (Mrazek & Haggerty, 1994), affirms that there is an existing pool of effective community-level preventive interventions and defines the gap as a problem in information dissemination. The goal is to improve the transfer of knowledge so that effective or model programs can be more effectively implemented.

Two alternative approaches go beyond the IOM model in the attempt to integrate research and practice. The first, the participatory action research approach (PAR), emphasizes the importance for all stakeholders–including researchers, practitioners, funders, participants, and advocates–to participate in the research process, formulate the research questions, and interpret and apply research findings (Green, 2001; Patton, 2002). The second, the social action research model, utilizes a methodology that integrates social change into the research process in a cyclic or spiral process. In contrast to the models discussed previously, the social action research model focuses on a process including identification of the problem, specification of program solutions, implementation, evaluation of the action, and eventual social change. Both of these models were utilized in Phase I and Phase II of the HFA Research Network. The goal of the next section is to summarize the Network's history in an effort to make recommendations for a systematic process of integrating science, practice, and research dissemination in future work.

FIGURE 1. Barriers and Bridges: Integrating Prevention Practice and Prevention Science

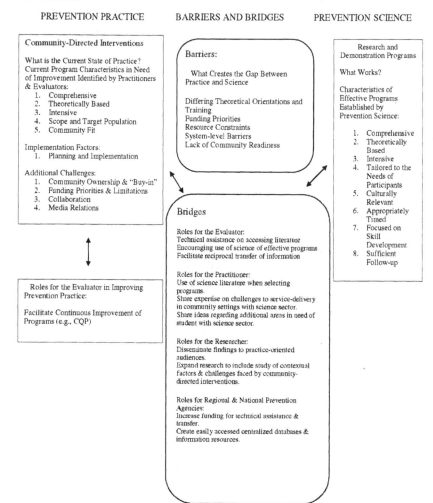

HISTORY OF RESEARCH NETWORK AND ORIGINAL GOALS

In 1994, PCA America launched the HFA Research Network to bring together two groups of researchers: academic researchers and community-based evaluators of HFA programs. The original goals were to: (a) improve the quantity and quality of HFA evaluated programs; (b) create a common database describing HFA programs, participants, and outcomes; (c) encourage secondary analyses of existing evaluative data; (d) develop more efficient methods to identify and engage families; (e) identify the most efficient and reliable methods for measuring participant change; (f) identify and address the critical unanswered questions inherent in documenting and enhancing program outcomes; and (g) over time, strengthen researcher-practitioner collaboration at the local, state, and national levels.

The Research Network itself was described as a unique experiment in how to build a knowledge base (Kahn, 1993) and has been viewed as a subject worthy of empirical study. By bringing together those conducting the most sophisticated program evaluations and those conducting quasi- and non-experimental designs in action settings, the Network has fostered a deeper understanding of the experience among its members, allowing the Research Network to provide guidance for others embarking on similar research collaborations (Daro & Harding, 1999). The Network's central role in developing the HFA's national computerized management information system and in completing the first-ever HFA national implementation study exemplifies the degree of collaboration (30 states participated in the former and almost 200 sites in 14 states in the latter) that has already been stimulated.

The HFA Research Network had two distinct phases. In Phase I, the entire constituency consisted of researchers: academic researchers and community-based evaluators of HFA programs. After 5 years, a consensus within the Research Network and external recommendations from the field converged, providing impetus for a new more inclusive Phase II. In Phase II, the Researcher Practitioner Council (RPC) was created, consisting of 25 researchers and 15 practitioners from across the country.

HFA Research Network Phase I (1994-1999)

From 1994-1999, 50 researchers from 25 states were active members. They were employed in state agencies, universities, and evaluation firms and they spanned the fields of child maltreatment, public health, and early childhood programs. Educational backgrounds included psychology, public health, child development, and social work. These rich and varied backgrounds ensured that no one theoretical orientation would dominate research questions or evaluation strategies, but they also represented barriers to being able to work together (as depicted in Figure 1). In the next section, we describe how the Research Network created an infrastructure for bridging these barriers. Specifically, the processes of developing common goals, shared decision-making, and building consensus were processes that proved useful.

Phase I processes. During the early years of the Network, PCA America helped to direct and nurture the Research Network. Nationally recognized experts (in child abuse, home visiting, and early childhood development) participated in the annual Network meetings. Committees were developed to work on the major goals that had been established (e.g., risk assessment, national database, outcomes and measurement issues, and research questions). Thus, the Network provided an infrastructure for promoting the bridging roles of evaluator, practitioner, and researcher. For example, researchers and evaluators shared the goal of emphasizing science as a basis for effective programs. Researchers made formal presentations as well as engaged in informal exchanges with practitioners during the committee meetings. The entire Network agreed upon decision-making processes that would allow the ongoing work of the individual committees to be debated and reviewed by Network members and consultants. The products developed in the individual committees were subject to review, and consensus was required before products designed to provide guidance to others were accepted and disseminated. The major accomplishments and products of the Research Network throughout Phases I and II are depicted in Table 1. The dominant foci of Phase I were to improve the quantity and quality of HFA evaluations and to create a common national database that would allow for comparability in describing HFA programs, participants, and outcomes. Other critical needs identified early on were the need for more efficient and reliable methods to identify and engage families and credible instruments for measuring participant change.

During Phase I, five annual meetings (1 to 3 days in duration) were convened, quarterly mailings on programmatic and policy development issues were instituted, conference calls were held, and two major research-practitioner roundtables were convened at the National PCA America conferences. The most significant Phase I initiative was a 3-year review of the data elements being used by all Healthy Families programs (30 state systems were included) in order to make recommendations for a national, computerized, management information system.

Phase I outcomes. Phase I was immensely successful in establishing a national researcher collaborative network and in transforming the network from a group of individual researchers to a collaborative that quickly developed a sense of shared mission. From the beginning, the network was characterized by shared ownership and collaborative leadership. Perhaps the most significant accomplishments were made in the areas of

TABLE 1. RPC Timetable of Transitions and Growth/Evolution

Phase I	Nat'l meetings	Task forces	Quarterly mailings	Nat'l research roundtables	Eval studies	3-yr data element study	PIMS	Outcome measures pool	4-yr Nat'l imp study	Special Issue on HFA
94	×	×				PLAN				
95	×	×	×	×		×				
96	×	×	×			×				
97	×	×	×	×		×	PIMS 1			
98	×	×	×							
99	×	×	×	×	17		PIMS 2			
Phase II	Nat'l meetings R&P					4-yr imp study				
00							PIMS 3			
01			×						×	
02							PIMS 4		×	
03			×				PIMS 5		×	PLAN
04					25				×	×
05										×

Goals (a) and (b), i.e., HFA evaluations and creating a common database. There was a significant increase in the quality and quantity of HFA evaluated programs. During Phase I, approximately 17 evaluations were completed and 18 additional studies were in progress. (Partnerships with university researchers were also formed to develop scientific evaluations and to conduct secondary analyses.) For example, a content analysis was conducted on the Family Stress Checklist (FSC) using data from 15 network studies. The most significant accomplishment of Phase I was the completion of a 3-year, 30-state review that informed the initial development of the computerized Program Information Management System and the Participant-Tracking components (PIMS I and II). These components were designed to supply information about HFA site resources, target communities, funding sources, and collaborating agencies, and to track participant characteristics as well as to evaluate the level and quality of services participants receive. PIMS established standard data elements that would allow HFA to collect more consistent evidence about program fidelity and program effectiveness.

The network also worked to develop more efficient methods to identify and engage families and to measure participant change. The network's deliberations and studies resulted in better delineation of the methodological challenges involved in operationalizing engagement, retention, and creative outreach as well as the challenges associated with engaging and retaining families. The research network also initiated a process of identifying measures that were psychometrically sound, user-friendly, and appropriate for measuring HFA program impacts. During the final 2 years of Phase I, improved definitions of these implementation processes were developed, and a pool of higher quality measures was identified. The work resulted in increased comparability across sites by encouraging common methods of risk assessment, common goal domains, and a pool of quality scientific outcome measures. (These definitions and measures were communicated to state Technical Assistants/Quality Assurance staff across the country for dissemination back to the programs.)

Several critical issues/challenges were identified as the funding for Phase I was about to end. Internally, the participants in the Research Network raised the following critical questions: How could network members coordinate the publication of findings? How could joint research projects be promoted and funded? How could HFA findings be best communicated among network members and the field at large?

In addition to these internally generated questions, external influences helped shaped the next phase in the development of the Research Network. In 1999, the most comprehensive national study of home visiting programs was conducted by The David and Lucile Packard Foundation. Several critical shortcomings were identified. Recommendations by the study's authors (Gomby, Culross, & Behrman, 1999) made it clear that home visiting programs and their national organizations should bring together researchers and practitioners in order to launch efforts to assess implementation fidelity and better understand and improve implementation and quality of services. This recommendation and the experience of the first 5 years of the network confirmed that a significant gap existed between research and practice and that it could be filled only by broadening the research network to include practitioners as full partners.

HFA Research Practice Network (RPN) Phase II (2000-2004)

The impetus for Phase II activities came from both internal and external sources. After five years of researchers and evaluators working closely together, it was clear that this group was not capable of closing the research-to-practice gap alone. Examinations of programs in substance abuse treatment, education, social service, community development, and virtually every other field reveal similar gaps (Schorr, 1997). For example, Lamb, Greenlick, and McCarty (1998) conducted a national study for the IOM focusing on the research-to-practice gap in the drug and alcohol abuse arena and identified strategies that can be used to close the gap. These strategies included researchers learning more about the complex organizational and community-level challenges required for successful dissemination, and practitioners receiving more training and education.

HFA also recognized the gap and the need to broaden the partnerships involved in promoting the HFA model. In 1999, the HFA Research Network consisted of 50 researchers in 33 states. A grant provided by the Packard Foundation allowed 25 of the original 50 researchers to join together with 15 practitioners from across the country in order to understand and grapple with contemporary research-to-practice issues and community concerns. The Researcher Practitioner Council (RPC) was born and the HFA Research Network was transformed into the Research Practice Network. The objectives of Phase II were to create a forum that would reflect and integrate research-practice issues. Moreover, with funding from the Packard and Gerber Foundations ($1 million and $300,000 grants, respectively), HFA responded to the recommendation made by the Packard Report (Gomby, Culross, & Behrman, 1999). That report recommended a "dedicated effort led by the field to improve the quality and implementation of existing home visiting programs..."(p. 24). PCA America and RPC accepted that challenge.

Phase II process. Building meaningful bridges between scientists and practitioners is a formidable challenge. Historically there have been far too few research-to-practice links, and each group has been socialized within a culture that contributes to misunderstanding. The goals of the RPC were derived, in part, from an awareness of the limitations of past research paradigms in the social and behavioral sciences, specifically: (a) the tendency to dichotomize research and practice, and devalue practitioners and "real world" researchers, (b) under-appreciation for the importance of integrating local knowledge with externally initiated intervention and research, and (c) inadequate concern about the sustainability of social interventions when external funding runs out. In fact, with science advancing so rapidly, it is understandably challenging for practitioners to stay abreast of scientific developments and their implications for evidence-based practice. It may be even more challenging for researchers to become fully aware of the administrative support needed to effectively integrate innovations into existing service delivery systems and to appreciate the complexities of the organizational change process. Having practitioners in the mix helps assure that the researchers formulate research/evaluation questions that are important to practitioners and reflective of what is happening on the ground.

Much of the RPC's first year was spent learning enough about the "other group" to allow an equality of collaboration. The research-to-practice collaboration that developed was and is an evolving process. The research agenda was decided in collaboration and guided by the needs of both the practice and research communities. Collaborative activities included exchanging resources and building two-way learning relationships. As the RPC moved into the tangible work of designing and implementing a national implementation study, the complementary expertise of both sets of partners and the complementary nature of the work became increasingly apparent. The fact that the work groups had to integrate issues relevant to practitioners with issues that could also contribute to prevention science required real bi-directional interactions and knowledge exchange. One outcome of the dialogue was an increasingly ecological understanding of the etiology of child maltreatment, one that emphasized parent-child interaction and the broader contexts of community and culture. Over time, the work of collaboration led to relationships based on mutual trust, respect for diversity in thinking, a willingness to collaborate in conducting and publishing research, increased ownership of research and evaluation findings, and an increased likelihood of acting on research and evaluation findings.

Phase II outcomes. The HFA Research Practice Network embarked on a 4-year national implementation study (Harding, Reid, Oshana, & Holton, 2004) aimed at informing the field about site characteristics, family retention, service intensity, service content, and staff retention. It was the focal point of Phase II and required most of the available time and resources. This study was a huge undertaking and the largest collaborative study of home visiting programs ever conducted. The study's architects included researchers and practitioners from 14 states, employing data from nine states and over 100 sites. Their three major objectives were fostering research-practice collaboration, implementing an evidence-based quality improvement strategy, and applying the knowledge gained throughout HFA and beyond (Harding, Reid, Oshana, & Holton, 2004). This study has provided the first comprehensive description of national implementation and identified factors associated with successful implementation. The RPC worked with HFA/PCA America to disseminate the findings of the Implementation Study and to use this information to develop recommendations that can guide future research and practice. A summary of the findings and lessons learned has been prepared and disseminated to HFA programs across the country. PCA America and the Research Practice Network are now in the process of designing interventions to enhance retention and implementation fidelity with the aim of better understanding the relationship between implementation and outcomes.

An ongoing focus of Phase II was continuing to improve the quantity and quality of evaluations of HFA programs. Both the number of evaluations and their size and scope grew considerably. There were 25 evaluations conducted during the 4-year Phase II period compared to the 17 of Phase I. Moreover, most of the evaluations conducted during Phase II were state-level or multi-site evaluations. The findings presented in the Harding, Galano, Martin, Huntington, and Schellenbach HFA outcomes review (see this issue) were based on 242 sites from 17 states and over 100 field-based evaluations. The work of collaborating in Phases I and II had a major impact on the willingness and the ability of researchers and practitioners to work together on the important tasks of evaluating HFA programs and preparing those evaluations for scholarly publications. The fact that so many network members were able to partner with practitioners, policymakers, and organizational leaders to generate scholarly publications for this volume reflects success in building critical bridges that did not exist before.

DISCUSSION

Kelly (2003) urged professionals in community psychology to foster social norms that encouraged ongoing dialogues among researchers, practitioners, and policymakers in order to strengthen the research-to-practice domain. This article chronicles the contributions of the HFA RPN, a unique 10-year partnership among researchers, practitioners, and policymakers in the field of child abuse prevention that exemplifies the approach advocated by Kelly. The following discussion addresses the RPN's attempt to integrate science, practice, and research and the challenges associated with supporting widespread dissemination. This discussion explains the impact of the RPN by examining three goals: (a) expanding knowledge on processes and outcomes of practitioner-scientist partnerships, (b) creating a common national database, and (c) formulating a research agenda of key questions in child abuse prevention.

Expanding Knowledge Base on Processes and Outcomes of Practitioner-Scientist Partnerships

The first goal was to build a knowledge base concerning the factors that facilitate and maintain practitioner-scientist partnerships within and across communities. The RPN focused specifically on efforts to improve the quantity and quality of HFA evaluations and programs. Much of the research conducted by RPN researchers has focused on successful collaboration among partners within community-based coalitions and groups rather than on conducting clinical trials. For example, with the growing awareness of the influence of the social context on individuals, families, and communities, much of this research has focused on qualitative analyses of selected partnerships (Green, 2001). HFA and the RPN need to take their research plan to the next level. In keeping with the recommendations by Butterfoss, Goodman, and Wandersman (1993), it may be productive, therefore, for HFA to focus on comparisons of more and less successful program sites to determine the factors that enhance coalition development and program implementation. Examples of successful sites could include the HFA site in New York, which has recently been distinguished as "a program that works" by the Rand Corporation (Mitchell-Herzfeld, Izzo, Greene, Lee, & Lowenfels, 2005). Other sites such as Arizona and Ohio/Kentucky (see this volume) showed considerable promise.

Unfortunately, significantly less research is available on diffusion of effective community-based partnerships across communities, states, and beyond. Hallfors (2002) determined that local prevention coalitions, such as HFP, function most effectively if (a) the team has clearly structured and focused goals, (b) they implement interventions that have a strong evidence base, and (c) there is a mechanism for providing ongoing proactive technical assistance. Factors that enhance the growth and sustainability of home visiting programs can be identified through research within HFA's nationwide research-practice network. In fact, several examples of bringing a program to scale at the local or state-level do exist in the RPN (Galano, Credle, Perry, Berg, Huntington, & Steif, 2001; Krysik & LeCroy and Ammerman et al., this volume). The article by Galano and colleagues (2001) documenting and analyzing the key elements involved in developing the

Hampton Healthy Families Partnership (HFP) and taking the program to scale is one example. Key elements included supportive political leadership, a collaborative budget, a collaborative structure for service delivery, a focus on system conversion, a universal approach, independent evaluation, new funding, a small steering committee of investors, champions, and a sense of urgency. After HFP went to scale, Galano and Huntington (2002) conducted the Benchmark Study, an empirical analysis of multiple community-based indicators of child and family well-being (such as rates of infant mortality and child abuse and neglect). The Hampton site outperformed all of the comparison communities, documenting the positive impact of prevention on measures of community-level health. (For a more complete summary, see Harding et al., this volume). Thus, Galano and Huntington provided additional evidence of the positive impact of voluntary prevention programs on community indices of a positive social environment. The body of research initiated through the RPN identified specific characteristics of community-based prevention programs that were determined to be successful in the process of replication and expansion. Carefully documented accounts that provide an understanding of the processes behind the changes that ultimately lead to improved outcomes in sustained prevention programs are in short supply, but they can provide valuable guidance for other communities across the country.

Creating a Common National Database
(The Program Information Management System)

The second goal of the HFA RPN was to create a common database for describing HFA program participants and outcomes, namely the Program Information Management System (PIMS). Linney (2005) emphasized that a network of coalitions could utilize a common set of indicators that would promote comparative analyses across sites. Scientists and practitioners each contribute a unique perspective on the effectiveness of prevention programs and community implementation. University researchers focus on the empirical foundation for identifying the effects of programs on risk and protective factors (Maton, Schellenbach, Leadbeater, & Solarz, 2005). Practitioners provide invaluable information on processes involved in the interaction of social context with program development and implementation. The RPN provided a rare coalition of community-based partnerships and researchers that allows for a better understanding of the real-world, system-level barriers, and ideas about what contextual factors need to be addressed in future implementation of prevention science in the community (see Harding et al., this volume). Eventually, the use of a common database will allow opportunities for meta-analyses and other methodologies that could better identify patterns of change. Such a system of measurement could then be utilized within the RPN to enhance program implementation. Research of this scope can occur only with programmatic efforts based on strong national leadership and federal financial support.

Consistent with the advice of Linney and other social scientists to develop a common set of measures, and as described briefly above, the HFA RPN developed a data collection system called PIMS. PIMS is a common database that encompasses data on participants, retention rates, prevention service delivery models, and specific program outcomes for sites across 30 states. HFA researchers have utilized PIMS to examine multiple outcomes such as child physical health, child development, quality of parenting, and reported rates of child abuse and neglect. By making this national data framework available to all HFA sites, the RPN has been instrumental in identifying factors that influence successful engagement and retention of HFA families. In fact, the common database provided the data for the national implementation study funded by the Packard and Gerber Foundations. Moreover, Harding, Reid, Oshana, and Holton (2004) reported that the *communal* work accomplished in Phase I of the Network resulted in increased comparability of standardized risk assessment procedures, mutually defined program goals, and a comparable pool of program outcomes across sites. In the subsequent Phase II, HFA RPN focused on examination of potential participant risk factors that may affect program engagement and retention. This domain of research would benefit from RPN sponsored university-community partnerships. The next phase of the research (Phase III) should focus on systematic research into the relationship between risk factors and ways in which programs can be modified to enhance engagement and retention. Research should also focus on national variability in risk level of clients at enrollment and the impact of client risk on patterns of engagement and retention.

Recent research by McCurdy and Daro (2001) and Olds et al. (1999) suggested that client enrollment and participation are influenced by factors at multiple levels of analysis including demographic factors like age and ethnicity, individual attributes of the parent, family or provider, or characteristics of the program or neighborhood. In subsequent research utilizing hierarchical linear modeling procedures to examine the contributions of participant characteristics, home visitor characteristics, and program characteristics, RPN researchers reported that home visitor and program characteristics accounted for one-third of variance in program duration (Daro, McCurdy, Falconnier, & Stojanovic, 2003). More specifically, clients who were older, unemployed, and enrolled earlier in their pregnancies were more likely to receive a greater number of services. Home visitors who were younger retained clients in the program for a longer period of time. This research represents an excellent example of a design that examines the interaction of multiple levels of analysis in an existing dataset.

Formulating a Research Agenda of Key Questions in Child Abuse Prevention

The third goal was to develop a research agenda consisting of key questions relevant to high-quality program evaluation and research as well to promote positive program development. One key question that has emerged from the work of the RPN focuses on the extent to which the variation in the types of research-practitioner partnerships is associated with variations in successful outcomes at the program site level. The manuscripts in this volume describing the growth of the home visiting programs in Arizona and Kentucky/Ohio provide important insights. Those sites spent considerable time forming their evaluations and developing strong evaluator-practitioner partnerships from the very beginning. Those evaluations contributed to quality improvement through continuous feedback. These states' systems have also been successful in achieving positive intermediate outcomes, preparing each initiative to go to scale statewide, and gradually employing increasingly rigorous evaluation methods. RPN's future research agenda should address four key questions. First, how successful are prevention coalitions in producing specified positive client outcomes? Second, when is it appropriate to bring the prevention coalition to scale? Third, if programs are taken to scale, how successful is the coalition in replicating and expanding the local program? And fourth, does the type of researcher-practitioner partnership mediate site success? For example, if a site fails to move slowly through the research process to strengthen the prevention coalition prior to moving to the measurement of program outcomes, as did the Alaska site (see Introduction, this issue), will the program be at risk in terms of financial support?

In fact, Linney (2005) asserts that although there is a substantial knowledge base regarding the types of community partnerships utilized across the country (e.g., the consultative-educational model, the expert-consulting model, and the university-community partnership model), little is known about the comparative effectiveness of these models. Research based on integrative, multi-level conceptual approaches rather than linear models tends to be more realistic in examining community-based prevention initiatives. For example, Wandersman and colleagues (2005) have developed a framework for summarizing the interaction of research, innovation development, and dissemination that prescribes the steps essential to dissemination of effective preventive innovations. Within the HFA network, the researchers were often the initiators of scientific testing of innovative home visitation programs. The HFA has produced multiple products such as journal articles, newsletters, conference presentations, and technical reports which were effective in translating knowledge into practitioner friendly tools for dissemination. The HFA RPN has provided examples of effective researcher-practitioner partnerships. However, more work is needed in terms of providing a leadership and funding infrastructure to maintain this innovative work in the field.

A second key question focuses on testing the utility of a social ecological approach to prevention/intervention efforts throughout the RPN. Much of the research concentrates rather narrowly on individual-level prevention/intervention efforts. In contrast, evidence indicates that prevention programs that are multidimensional and multi-level tend to be the most effective (Durlak, 1997). In this light, other research on home visitation prevention efforts has focused on identifying the characteristics of clients and their families that may affect program enrollment, retention, and ultimately, client outcomes. Shifting to the neighborhood and community level of analysis, research suggests that the social environment influences rates of client participation and engagement in voluntary prevention programs. Mothers who were isolated from friends and family and who resided in communities characterized by poor community health were significantly less likely to participate in home visiting programs compared to mothers who did not live in socially impoverished environments (McGuigan, Katzev, & Pratt, 2003). Once mothers were enrolled in a home visitation program, however, the impoverished mothers received more home visits compared to non-impoverished mothers.

In contrast, the research of Daro et al. (see this volume) which sampled 182 census blocks in six states, determined that parents living in the most distressed communities received more home visits. Daro's research represents an excellent exemplar of the role that the RPN has played in providing an infrastructure for multilevel prevention research.

These two studies, which go beyond the level of the individual, yield a more nuanced understanding of how people enter and remain in home visiting programs. Isolation and neighborhood distress may prevent many families from accessing services in the first place but, once enrolled, families receive more home visits. The findings from these studies suggest that future research must focus on the interaction of the social context and client, provider, and program characteristics. This ecological focus is especially critical for community-based prevention programs such as those implemented in the HFA network.

INTEGRATING PREVENTION POLICY
WITH PREVENTION RESEARCH AND PRACTICE

Prevention programs that target the individual, family, and community levels and also address social norms and public policy are likely to produce the most positive and sustained results (Durlak, 1997). The national variation in sites within the network presents the opportunity to examine characteristics of multi-level programs that are successful, particularly those that examine interactions among levels of social context. This type of research is sophisticated, however, and typically not possible without federal support and/or university partners. Indeed, the best models of practice-research collaboration reflect successful partnerships between researchers and practitioners. In 1998, the Institute of Medicine produced a report that summarized the gap between science and effective treatment of substance abuse disorders (Lamb, Greenlick, & McCarty, 1998). Despite great strides in research, the substance abuse treatment system in 1998 was indistinguishable from the one in place in 1975 (Sorensen, Guydish, Rawson, & Zweben, 2003). Following the report, the National Institute of Drug Abuse launched an initiative designed to blend research and practice, significantly benefiting both researchers and practitioners. There is a similar need for significant federal leadership in the child abuse and neglect arena.

The HFA RPN has also learned much from its experiences during the past 10 years. There is an urgent need to develop a long-term plan (5-10 years) to build a practice research collaborative to guide this work in the future. Based on the lessons learned from the previous 10 years of collaboration, the following ideas appear critical to the success and growth of the RPN and its impact on the field of community-based child abuse prevention research.

Preliminary Ideas for the HFA RPN Future Plan

Research-to-practice collaboration is an ongoing, long-term, and evolving process. The progress made during the first 10 years of the RPN is heartening. However, sustained progress requires more permanent structure and support. The circumstances that contribute to child abuse and neglect are long-standing. Meaningful solutions necessitate that PCA

America and the RPN stay the course and implement a long-term plan. Over the next 5 to 10 years, there are a number of important steps that the HFA Research Center should take to institutionalize the research-to-practice collaborations that have been established and to increase the rate at which prevention science is incorporated into child abuse and neglect prevention efforts in our communities.

1. Establish a long-term leadership and a formal structure to continue and grow the HFA RPN.

Although much has been accomplished during the past 10 years of work, the continuation of the research-practitioner partnerships within the HFA RPN requires a long-term plan. The collective talents and energy of the members of the RPN represent an invaluable resource which requires long-term support to attain its national goals in the future. The goals of the HFA RPN are (1) to assess the present state of the best science on child abuse prevention research, practice, and policy; (2) to plan initiatives that integrate research, practice, and policy on the prevention of child abuse and neglect; (3) to become the national center of child abuse prevention efforts within the HFA network and beyond; and (4) to create a structure for dissemination of the best science on child abuse prevention to the practice and policy arena. The work of the RPN has gained some real momentum; however, fiscal uncertainty and a lack of resources can undermine commitment and optimism. Designing multi-level, multi-state applied research takes time, and ensuring that scientific knowledge and innovations affect practice takes time and long-term federal and foundation support.

2. Strengthen and expand the researcher-practitioner partnerships and develop strong collaborations with policymakers and funding sources at the national, state, and local levels.

The Institute of Medicine (Lamb, Greenlick, & McCarty, 1998) and others recommend continuing to move from thinking in terms of research-practice to research-practice-policy. Based on this recommendation, it is critical that the planning of child abuse prevention initiatives be based on partnerships with policymakers and funding sources at the federal, state, and local levels. The exemplary work of Sorensen and colleagues in the field of substance abuse prevention provides a model for such successful collaboration.

3. Develop broad partnerships, joint ownership, and collaborative leadership.

The ongoing work of the collaboration can benefit from multiple partners who share a collective responsibility in the work of preventing child abuse and neglect. Stakeholders may come from numerous state or federal agencies and foundations. Their ownership of the mission and direct support of the work required is invaluable to the positive outcomes of the initiative.

4. *Further the use of evidence-based and useful prevention approaches/ interventions.*

The RPN should develop a Program Advisory Committee that recommends changes to community-based programs based on evidence-based standards. For example, PCA America has produced a recent summary of evidenced-based practice in home visitation research, "Evidenced-Based Practice at a Glance." Such a committee would be in a position to link with government and non-profit research-based centers and develop partnerships with universities and regional centers.

5. *Better integrate the work of RPN with HFA's dissemination and training.*

The value of scientific research should not be judged by the quality of the scholarly publication in which it appears, but by the broad dissemination of the information to frontline decision makers who are charged with delivering and improving day-to-day services. HFA's dissemination and training staff understand this gap between research and practice and need to be intimately involved in supporting widespread dissemination and adoption.

CONCLUSIONS

Unlike university-based clinical trials, community-driven prevention efforts are "owned" by service providers in the community. Building upon this understanding, the HFA RPN is demonstrating the benefits of researchers' and practitioners' collaboration to advance the field of child abuse and neglect prevention science. Today, the barriers between prevention science and prevention practice are better understood, as are the bridges to decrease the gap. Researchers, practitioners, and policymakers recognize that effective community-based prevention efforts can be effective in improving the quality of well-being for children and their parents. Yet, our science has generally not focused on understanding community-based efforts, and our policies have often lagged behind in creating resources to address these pressing issues. Now, we urgently need leadership and funding at the national level to enable regional and national prevention agencies, practitioners, scientists and evaluators to achieve their collective potential.

PCA America created the framework for this multi-state collaboration. That collaboration was not an end in itself, but a means to research that is capable of informing us about how to improve child abuse and neglect prevention programs. The papers in this volume demonstrate the impact of community-based approaches for improving the lives of children and parents. Together, they present a strong body of evidence concerning the effectiveness of researcher-practitioner partnerships in community-based child abuse prevention as well as policy directions that are required to bolster these efforts in the future. As underscored in the work of Margaret Mead in the introduction to this volume, "Never doubt that a small group of thoughtful, committed citizens can change the world." Indeed, collectively, they make a case for the impact of community-based research in child abuse prevention and present a call for action to focus on these directions in the next five years.

AUTHORS' NOTE

The authors would like to express their gratitude to the Carnegie, Packard, and Gerber Foundations for their support of the RPN and acknowledge those individuals who came together from across the country, bound only by their collective commitment to contribute to the knowledge base on child abuse and neglect prevention.

Robert Ammerman, OH	Richard Chase, MN	Thomas Gordon, FL
Elizabeth Anisfeld, NY	Debbie Cheatham, OH	Beth Green, OR
Juanita Arnold, FL	Margaret Clark, OH	Rose Greene, NY
Jose Ashford, AZ	Meredith Clay, CT	Joy Griffith, NY
Barbara Barrett, VA	Peggy Coffey, CT	Neil Guterman, NY
Dorothy Baum, NY	Perle Slavik Cowen, IA	Judith Hanley, VA
Carolyn Bivona, SC	Julie Crouch, IL	Michele Hansen, AK
Tim Black, CT	Anne Culp, OK	Kathryn Harding, HFA
Anne Brady, MA	Deborah Daro, HFA	John Heck, NY
Moshe Braner, VT	Javier Diaz, HFA	John K. Holton, HFA
Gail Breakey, HI	Sue Diehl, CT	Elizabeth Holtzapple, AZ
Elsbeth Brown, SC	Anne Duggan, HI	Lee Huntington, VA
Debra Caldera, AK	Linda Dunphy, VA	Rhonda Impink, IN
Linda Cameron, AK	Carla Edwards, FL	Fritz Jenkins, OR
Lynn Cannady, CA	James Elicker, IN	Elizabeth Jones, HFA
Sharon Carnahan, FL	Jerome Evans, CA	LaVohn Josten, MN
Terry Carrilio, CA	Lori Friedman, HFA	Beth Kapsch, OR
Janet Ceasar, PA	Joseph Galano, VA	Aphra Katzev, OR
Julie Chambliss, GA	Thomas Gannon, OH	Ann Keim, WI

Phyllis Kikendall, IN
Donna D. Klagholz, VA
Kerry Kriener-Althen, TN
John Landsverk, CA
Craig LeCroy, AZ
Carl Maas, SC
Karin MacKinnon, VA
Juliette Mackin, OR
Joanne Martin, IN
Sally S. Martin, NV
Courtney McAfee, GA
Karen McCurdy, HFA
Beth McDaid, PA
William McGuigan, OR
Gary Melton, SC
Kristin Mena, IN

Gail Meyers, TN
Joel Milner, IL
'Susan Mitchell-Herzfeld, NY
Carmel Munroe, FL
Judith Myers-Walls, IN
Carnot Nelson, FL
Ismail Noor, MI
Erin Oldham, ME
Domarina Oshana, HFA
Barbara Palmer, VA
Virginia Peckham, PA
Bingham Pope, TN
Clara Pratt, OR
Frank Putnam, OH
Virginia Rauh, NY
Robert Reid, HFA

Richard Roberts, UT
Kira Rodriguez, AK
Jaylene Krieg Schaefer, OH
Cynthia Schellenbach, MI
Betty Shiels, KY
Thomas K. Smith, PA
Mary Steir, CT
Kathleen Strader, MI
Darcy Strouse, VA
Karen T. Thompkinson, MD
Mary Trankel, MT
Ching-Tung Wang, HFA
Kate Whitaker, AZ
Judith Williams, FL
Carolyn Winje, HFA
Carla Woodson, NJ

REFERENCES

American Association for Protecting Children (1988). *Highlights of official child neglect and abuse reporting–1986.* Denver, CO: American Humane Association.

Baker, A., Piotrkowski, C. S., & Brooks-Gunn, J. B. (1999). The Home Instruction Program for Preschool Youngsters (HIPPY). *The Future of Children, 9,* 116-133.

Baker, T., David, S., & Soucy, G. (Eds.) (1995). *Reviewing the behavioral science knowledge base on technology transfer.* Washington, DC: National Institute of Drug Abuse.

Belsky, J. (1980). Child maltreatment: An ecological integration. *American Psychologist, 35,* 320-335.

Butterfoss, F. D., Goodman, R. M., & Wandersman, A. (1993). Community coalitions for health promotion and disease prevention. *Health Education Research: Theory and Practice, 8*(3), 315-330.

Cicchetti, D., & Lynch, M. (1993). Towards an ecological/transactional model of community violence and child maltreatment: Consequences for children's development. In D. Scharff (Ed.), *Children and violence* (pp. 96-118). New York: Guilford Press.

Cicchetti, D., & Toth, S. L. (2000). Child maltreatment in the early years of life. In J. D. Osofsky & H. E. Fitzgerald (Eds.), *WAIMH Handbook of Infant Mental Health, Vol. 4: Infant mental health in groups at high-risk* (pp. 255-294). New York: Cambridge University Press.

Daro, D. A. (1996). *Building community capacity to prevent child abuse.* Chicago: The National Committee for Prevention of Child Abuse.

Daro, D. A. (2000). *Public opinion and behaviors regarding child abuse prevention: 1999 survey.* Chicago: Prevent Child Abuse America.

Daro, D. A., & Cohn-Donnelly, A. (2002). Child abuse and prevention: Accomplishments and challenges. In J. Myers et al. (Eds.), *The APSAC handbook on child maltreatment* (2nd ed., pp. 431-448). Newbury Park, CA: Sage.

Daro, D. A., & Harding, K. A. (1999). Healthy Families America: Using research to enhance practice. *The Future of Children, 9,* 152-176.

Daro, D. A., McCurdy, K., Falconnier, L., & Stojanovic, D. (2003). Sustaining new parents in home visitation services; Key participant and program factors. *Child Abuse and Neglect, 27,* 1101-1125.

Durlak, J. (1997). *Successful prevention programs for children and adolescents.* New York: Plenum.

Elias, M. J. (1997). Reinterpreting dissemination of prevention programs as widespread implementation with effectiveness and fidelity. In G. R. Adams (Ed.), *Establishing prevention services* (pp. 253-289). Thousand Oaks, CA: Sage.

Galano, J., Credle, W., Perry, D., Berg, S., Huntington, L., & Steif, E. (2001). Developing and sustaining a successful community prevention initiative: The Hampton Healthy Families Partnership, 495-509.

Galano, J., & Huntington, L. (2002). *FY 2002 Healthy Families Partnership Benchmark Study: Measuring community-wide impact.* Prepared by the Applied Social Psychology Research Institute, College of William and Mary, Williamsburg, VA.

Garbarino, J., & Barry, F. (1997). The community context of child abuse and neglect. In J. Eckenrode (Ed.), *Understanding abusive families: An ecological approach to theory and practice* (pp. 56-85). San Francisco, CA: Jossey-Bass.

Gomby, D. S., Culross, P. L., & Behrman, R. E. (1999). Home visiting: Recent program evaluations–Analysis and recommendations. *The Future of Children, 9*(1), 4-26.

Government Accounting Office (GAO) (1990). Home Visiting: A promising early intervention strategy for at-risk families. GAO/HRD-90-83. Washington, DC: Author.

Green, L. W. (2001). From research to "best practices" in other settings and populations. *American Journal of Health Behavior Research, 25,* 165-178.

Green, L. W. (2002). *Best practices from other fields of prevention research: What can child abuse prevention learn.* Paper presented at the Imagine a Nation Without Child Abuse: Combing our Strengths for Prevention Conference, Dallas, TX.

Green, L. W., Daniel, M., & Novick, L. (2001). Partnerships and coalitions for community-based research. *Public Health Reports, 116*(Suppl. 1), 20-30.

Green, L. W., & Johnson, J. L. (1996, November-December). Dissemination and utilization of health promotion and disease prevention knowledge: Theory, research, and experience. *Canadian Journal of Public Health,* S11-S17.

Hallfors, D., Cho, H., Livert, D., & Kadushin, C. (2002). Fighting back against substance abuse: Are community coalitions winning? *American Journal of Preventive Medicine, 23,* 237-245.

Harding, K., Reid, R., Oshana, D., & Holton, J. (2004). Initial results of the National Healthy Families America implementation study: A report submitted to the David and Lucille Packard Foundation. Chicago, IL: Prevent Child Abuse America.

Israel, B. A., Schulz, A. J., Parker, A. E., & Becker, A. B. (1998). Review of community-based research: Assessing partnership approaches to improve public health. *Annual Review of Public Health, 19,* 173-202.

Kahn, R. (1993). *An experiment in scientific organization: The MacArthur Foundation program in mental health and human development.* Chicago: The MacArthur Foundation.

Kelly, J. G. (2003). Science and community psychology: Social norms for pluralistic inquiry. *American Journal of Community Psychology, 31*(3-4), 213-217.

Kempe, C. H., Silverman, F. N., Steele, B. F., Drogemueller, W., & Silver, H. K. (1962). The battered child syndrome. *Journal of the American Medical Association, 62,* 100-110.

Kendall-Tackett, K. A., Williams, L. M., & Finkelhor, D. (1993). Impact of sexual abuse on children: A review and synthesis of recent empirical studies. *Psychological Bulletin, 113,* 164-180.

Lamb, S., Greenlick, M. R., & McCarty, D. (Eds.) (1998). *Bridging the gap between practice and research: Forging partnerships with community-based drug and alcohol treatment.* Washington, DC: National Academy Press.

Linney, J. A. (2005). Might we practice what we've preached? Thoughts on the special issue papers. *American Journal of Community Psychology, 35* (3-4), 253-258.

Maton, K. I., Schellenbach, C. J., Leadbeater, J., & Solarz, A. L. (2005). *Investing in children, youth, families, and communities: Strengths-based research and policy.* Washington, DC: American Psychological Association.

McCurdy, K., & Daro, D. (2001). Parent involvement in family support programs: An integrated theory. *Family Relations, 50,* 113-121.

McGuigan, W. M., Katzev, A. R., & Pratt, C. (2003). Multi-level determinants of mothers' engagement in home visitation services. *Family Relations, 52,* 271-278.

Mitchell-Herzfeld, S., Izzo, C., Greene, R., Lee, E., & Lowenfels, A. (2005). Evaluation of Healthy Families New York (HFNY): First year program impacts. Rensselaer, NY: New York State Office of Children and Family Services, Bureau of Evaluation and Research, Albany, NY: Center for Human Services Research, University at Albany.

Morrissey, E., Wandersman, A., Seybolt, D., Nation, M., Crusto, C., & Davino, K. (1997). Toward a framework for bridging the gap between science and practice in prevention. *Evaluation and Program Planning, 20,* 367-377.

Mrazek, P. J., & Haggerty, R. J. (Eds.) (1994). *Reducing risks for mental disorders: Frontiers for preventive intervention research.* Washington, DC: National Academy Press.

National Institute of Mental Health (1998). *Priorities for prevention research at NIMH: A report of the National Advisory Mental Health Council Workgroup on Mental Disorders Prevention Research* (NIMH Publication No. 98-4321). Washington, DC: US Government Printing Office.

National Research Council and Institute of Medicine (2000). *From neurons to neighborhoods: The science of early childhood* development (J. P. Shonkoff & D. A. Phillips, Eds.). Washington, DC: National Academy Press.

Olds, D. L., Henderson, C. R., Kitzman, H. J., Eckenrode, J., Cole, R., & Tatelbaum, R. (1999). Prenatal and infancy home visitation by nurses: Recent findings. *The Future of Children, 9,* 44-66.

Patton, M. Q. (2002). A conversation with Michael Quinn Patton. *Harvard Family Research Project, 8,* 10-11.

Schorr, L. (1997). *Common purpose.* New York: Simon & Schuster.

Schorr, L. (2002). The role of evidence in improving outcomes for children. In C. Bruner (Ed.), *Funding what works: Exploring the role of research on the effective programs ad practices in government decision-making* (pp. 1-6). Des Moines, IA: National Center for Service Integration.

Sedlack, A. J., & Broadhurst, D. D. (1996). *Third National Incidence Study of Child Abuse and Neglect.* National Center on Child Abuse and Neglect, Washington, DC: US Department of Health and Human Services.

Sorensen, J. L., Rawson, R. A., Guydish, J., & Zweben, J. E. (Eds.) (2003). *Drug abuse treatment through collaboration: Practice and research participants that work.* Washington, DC: American Psychological Association.

Tricket, P., Kurtz, D. A., & Pizzigati, K. (2005). Resilient outcomes in abused and neglected children: Bases for strengths-based intervention and prevention policies. In K. Matton, C. Schellenbach, B. Leadbeater, & A. Solarz (Eds.), *Investing in children, youth, families, and communities: Strengths-based research and policy* (p. 73-96). Washington, DC: American Psychological Association.

Tricket, P., & McBride-Chang, C. (1995). The developmental impact of different forms of child abuse and neglect. *Developmental Review, 15,* 311-337.

Wandersman, A., Flaspohler, P., & Saul, J. (2005). *Dissemination/implementation issues in effective child maltreatment prevention and youth violence prevention.* Unpublished manuscript. Washington, DC: American Psychological Association.

Wandersman, A., & Florin, P. (2003). Community interventions and effective prevention. *American Psychologist, 58,* 441-448.

Widom, C. S. (1989). Does violence beget violence? A critical examination of the literature. *Psychological Bulletin, 106,* 3-28.

US Advisory Board on Child Abuse and Neglect (1990). *Child abuse and neglect: Critical first steps in responding to a national emergency* (1st Report). Washington, DC: US Department of Health and Human Services, US Government Printing Office.

US Advisory Board on Child Abuse and Neglect (1993). *The continuing child protection emergency: A challenge to the nation* (3rd Report). Washington, DC: US Department of Health and Human Services, US Government Printing Office.

US Department of Health and Human Services (2000). *Healthy People 2010* (Conference edition, in two volumes). Washington, DC: US Department of Health and Human Services.

US Department of Health and Human Services (2003). Administration on Children, Youth and Families, *Child Maltreatment 2001.* Washington, DC: U.S. Government Printing Office.

doi:10.1300/J005v34n01_03

Healthy Families America®
State Systems Development:
An Emerging Practice to Ensure
Program Growth and Sustainability

Lori Friedman
Lisa Schreiber

Prevent Child Abuse America

SUMMARY. In an era of fiscal constraints and increased accountability for social service programs, having a centralized and efficient infrastructure is critical. A well-functioning infrastructure helps a state reduce duplication of services, creates economies of scale, coordinates resources, supports high-quality site development and promotes the self-sufficiency and growth of community-based programs. Throughout the Healthy Families America home visitation network, both program growth and contraction have been managed by in-state collaborations, referred to as "state systems." This article explores the research base that supports the rationale for implementing state systems, describes the evolution of

Address correspondence to: Lori Friedman, MPH, Senior Prevention Analyst or Lisa Schreiber, AM, Director of HFA State Systems, Prevent Child Abuse America, 500 North Michigan Avenue, Suite 200, Chicago, IL 60611. (E-mail: lfriedman@prevent childabuse.org or lschreiber@preventchildabuse.org). Additional information and resources pertaining to Healthy Families America can be found on the website located at (www.healthyfamiliesamerica.org).

[Haworth co-indexing entry note]: "Healthy Families America® State Systems Development: An Emerging Practice to Ensure Program Growth and Sustainability." Friedman, Lori, and Lisa Schreiber. Co-published simultaneously in *Journal of Prevention & Intervention in the Community* (The Haworth Press, Inc.) Vol. 34, No.1/2, 2007, pp. 67-87; and: *The Healthy Families America® Initiative: Integrating Research, Theory and Practice* (ed: Joseph Galano) The Haworth Press, 2007, pp. 67-87. Single or multiple copies of this article are available for a fee from The Haworth Document Delivery Service [1-800-HAWORTH, 9:00 a.m. - 5:00 p.m. (EST). E-mail address: docdelivery@haworthpress.com].

state systems for Healthy Families America, and discusses the benefits, challenges and lessons learned of utilizing a systems approach. doi:10.1300/ J005v34n01_04 *[Article copies available for a fee from The Haworth Document Delivery Service: 1-800-HAWORTH. E-mail address: <docdelivery@ haworthpress.com> Website: <http://www.HaworthPress.com> © 2007 by The Haworth Press, Inc. All rights reserved.]*

KEYWORDS. Home visiting, infrastructure, program replication, state systems, sustainability, systems development

ENSURE PROGRAM GROWTH AND SUSTAINABILITY

Without sustainability, program effectiveness is of little consequence. Many interrelated issues contribute to the maintenance and growth of a program. The state systems that have evolved to support the Healthy Families America program provide useful examples of how the establishment of this type of infrastructure contributes to the strength and longevity of a program. This article describes the evolution of this process, highlights several theoretical frameworks these systems are building upon, and provides practical suggestions for state level planners interested in developing similar systems.

EVOLUTION OF HEALTHY FAMILIES AMERICA STATE SYSTEMS

In 1976, a home visiting program called Healthy Start was launched in Hawaii. Early program evaluations demonstrated encouraging results in the area of child abuse prevention. Based on this evidence, Prevent Child Abuse America (PCA America; formerly the National Committee to Prevent Child Abuse [NCPCA]) decided in 1992 to replicate this program on the U.S. mainland. Implementation began with 25 sites scattered throughout the country. Increased awareness of the short- and long-term impacts of child abuse, coupled with the availability of additional funding through resources such as Temporary Assistance to Needy Families (TANF) and tobacco settlement funds in the mid-1990s, enabled many states to implement multiple programs concurrently. By 1995, it became clear that skyrocketing program growth would quickly outstrip the capacity of the national office to provide training and technical assistance and, therefore, each state should "take responsibility for the well-being of all their children... by creating a permanent infrastructure that can support all children" (NCPCA, 1995, p. 5). At that time, with the support of the Freddie Mac Foundation, PCA America began devoting significant resources towards assisting states in the creation of planning teams or task forces that engaged state level administrators and policymakers in the growth of the Healthy Families America (HFA) program. In 1996, the need to provide more structure around the program with regard to quality implementation had emerged and became the catalyst for the creation of the credentialing process (See Appendix A). By 1997, a priority of the NCPCA was "to establish national and state capacity to build upon and expand existing service networks and provide expertise to local communities," leading to the formalization of the state systems department at the national level in 1998 (NCPCA, 1997, p. 2).

A goal of this department was to establish national and state capacity to expand existing service networks and provide expertise to local communities. With input from state-level leadership, a framework was developed to describe the primary activities of a state system by which to support the work of programs across the country. The framework suggests that there are 10 components or functional areas that contribute to a state's HFA or home visiting infrastructure. These areas include: (a) administration/governance, (b) strategic planning, (c) training and technical assistance, (d) community planning/site development, (e) continuous quality improvement/credentialing, (f) public relations/media, (g) public policy/advocacy, (h) collaboration, (i) public education (awareness)/outreach, and (j) communication (PCA America, 2001). The existence of these systems has enabled the program to evolve into a robust network of home visiting programs providing services to families in more than 400 communities (Diaz, Oshana, & Harding, 2004).

There is considerable variability among and between state systems. These systems have emerged for a variety of reasons and in a number of different ways. Data regularly collected at the site and state level by PCA America highlight the multiple ways in which systems are structured (Diaz et al., 2004; PCA America, 2003a; Schreiber & Friedman, 2004). Most systems are HFA-specific although a few states have systems that are inclusive of the range of home visiting programs operating throughout the state. Each state has reached a different developmental level based on their resources, needs and political environment. Some have a system of coordination primarily around one or two key functions such as training or quality assurance. Others are comprehensive and entirely centralized to the point that funding streams are blended and a statewide coordinator oversees all systems-related activities. The scope and structure of several HFA state systems have been described in the *Healthy Families America State Systems Development Guide:*

> "In Indiana, we consider our support of the Healthy Families program an important investment in our children and our future," said former Governor Kernan. We're extremely proud to be one of the leading states in the development of a central system to support individual Healthy Families programs around the state. Healthy Families Indiana ties everything together so that each site can best serve the families and children in their area, strengthen families and communities, and save lives. (PCA America, 2003b, p. 5)

The next phase in the evolution of support provided to the HFA network came via the creation of the Regional Resource Centers. Launched by PCA America in 2003, these centers work at the local, state, and regional levels to ensure that programs have the capacity to continue serving families by brokering that resources and developing new strategies to deliver services, such as distance learning trainings. To date, nearly every state with more than one HFA site has some infrastructure in place at the state level supported by either PCA America or a Regional Resource Center (PCA America, 2003a).

THEORETICAL BACKGROUND

As successful social programs attempt to replicate their models and bring them "to scale," infrastructure becomes an essential component of program development. Researchers in an article entitled the "Dissemination of Prevention Programs" concluded that infrastructures are needed to facilitate connections among program settings, innovators and experts as prevention programs are disseminated (Weissberg, Gullotta, Hampton, Ryan, & Adams, 1997).

A diverse body of research describes the characteristics found in successfully implemented programs (Backer, 1991; Backer, 2000; Mihalic, Irwin, Fagan, Ballard, & Elliott, 2004; Morrissey et al., 1997; Rogers, 1983; Rogers, 1995; Rogers & Kinkaid, 1981). Many of these characteristics are related to having an infrastructure to support the growth and sustainability of social service programming. In particular, the research on *diffusion of innovation* (Backer, 1995; Green, 2001; Rogers, 1983) and *program replication* (Bruner, 1996; Mihalic et al.; Morrissey et al.; Schorr, 1997) lends helpful frameworks that authenticate the need for and role of systems in program development.

Diffusion of Innovation

Diffusion of innovation research offers a framework to explore questions of systems reform and the institutionalization of social service programs. A leading researcher in this area, Rogers (1983) defines diffusion as "the process by which an innovation is communicated through certain channels over time among the members of a social system" (p. 5). This body of research is composed of four core elements: (a) the innovation itself (e.g., the program model being implemented, i.e., HFA); (b) the communication channels (e.g., the vehicles and opportunities created to enhance mutual sharing of resources and facilitate collaborative planning that lead to the implementation and sustainability of the program); (c) the time from exposure to adoption (e.g., the period of time from program planning to implementation and sustainability); and (d) the social system (e.g., evidence of political support that contributes to the sustainability of the program). The presence of an infrastructure such as the state systems created around the HFA program helps to contribute to the diffusion of this process.

Green (2001) and Backer (1995) argue the caveats of dissemination of knowledge and innovation. Green looks at the issue from the perspective of the application of *best practices* and the ability to generalize the impact of best practices to different contexts. Backer generates his theory from the field of *technology transfer* and the bridging of the gap between research and practice. Both researchers argue that static distribution of information is not enough. Dissemination requires the strategic sharing of information about programs and best practices with individuals, organizations and communities to enable them to create positive changes for society (Backer, 1991; Rogers, 1995). Information about programmatic best practices needs to be coupled with the provision of technical assistance and other resources to help ensure successful implementation and adoption (Backer, 2000; Mihalic et al., 2004; Morrissey et al., 1997). Ideally this support is formalized to maximize consistency and quality. At the national level, the leaders of HFA recognized that even intensive and ongoing training on the model would not be enough to ensure the quality and fidelity of the program. This led to the development of state systems that provide ongoing technical assistance, supervision, quality assurance and regular skills development opportunities (NCPCA, 1995).

Program Replication

Another area of research that authenticates state systems development is the literature on *program replication*, particularly the work of Schorr (1997) and Bruner (1996). In general, this work is concerned with how promising approaches to helping children and families can be successfully and appropriately replicated.

Schorr (1997) learned that growing programs "combine the replication of the essence of a successful intervention with the adaptation of many of its components to a new setting" (p. 60). As Schorr explains, the planners of a successful replication decide which components of the replication should be centralized and which should be individualized to local needs. This is the same philosophy HFA embraced when developing its initial program model. Inherent in these *critical elements* is a great deal of flexibility that allows communities to customize the program to meet their needs. For example, a critical element on service content states "services should focus on supporting the parent as well as supporting parent-child interaction and child development" (PCA America, 2004a, p. 54). HFA does not mandate one specific method for sites to provide this support, such as a specific program curriculum for parent education. Instead, individual states and programs decide what curriculum best meets the needs of the families they serve in a particular community. The flexibility inherent in the critical elements contributes to wide variation in program outcomes. Harding, Galano, Huntington, Martin, and Schellenbach (this volume) offer a further discussion of this issue.

Through her analysis of various case studies, Schorr (1997) details the following "elements of successful replications" (pp. 59-63): (a) the continuous backing of an intermediary organization offering expertise, outside support, legitimization and clout to help sustain the scaled-up intervention; (b) the importance of the system's institutional context (being aware of how institutional environment can influence practice); (c) the importance of the people context (that the individuals working on the replication are invested in the program); (d) an outcomes orientation to judge success; and (e) the addressing, directly and strategically, of the obstacles to large-scale change.

An application of Schorr's (1997) work is demonstrated by successful state systems that (a) operate through a work group or independent collaborative (the intermediary organization), (b) understand the political and social context within which the state system is being formed via advocacy and public policy functions, (c) engage and regularly communicate with staff and stakeholders involved with the program, (d) evaluate success through data collection and research, and (e) strategically plan growth and direction.

The work of Bruner (1996) reinforces Schorr's findings in her program replication research and moves the discussion toward systems reform issues. Bruner found four themes in systems reform efforts that have relevance for state systems development:

1. *Community-based*: Community level decision-making requires novel governance, management, and relationships between state and local entities;
2. *Holistic*: Systems are expected to deliver a seamless approach to families. Such a system mandates a new level of collaboration and communication;
3. *Results-accountable*: In the movement towards outcomes, a systematic manner of collecting concrete results is critical;
4. *Participatory*: In a move to make a system more inclusive, broad-based strategies must be developed to engage a wide variety of consumers and constituents.

Taken together, the work of Schorr and Bruner helps build the case for state systems development by emphasizing the importance of a responsive entity that understands and addresses the sociopolitical environment when bringing together a variety of innovations to create a system of services for children and families.

Research has also been conducted in the fields of violence prevention and substance abuse prevention to determine the critical factors associated with successful program implementation and replication. These factors include the need for effective organizational support (which includes administrative support, agency stability, having a shared vision and interagency links), having skilled, flexible and motivated staff with relevant expertise, and providing a strong, proactive package of training and technical assistance (Mihalic et al., 2004; Morrissey et al., 1997).

As HFA state systems have evolved, they are addressing many of these critical factors. The credentialing process at both the site and the multisite levels helps to ensure that there is adequate support available to facilitate program implementation and sustainability. In addition, many states have systems evolved to the point that there are dedicated individuals responsible for securing funding, providing leadership to create and maintain a shared vision, and nurturing relationships with partners across the state. State systems have proved invaluable in establishing communication pathways such as having regular meetings, operating listservs and providing technical assistance conference calls in which problem-solving among and between program staff at various sites can occur. This contributes to the development of new skills and helps minimize staff frustration and turnover (Innovative Strategies: Staff Retention, n.d.; Salus, 2004; U.S. Department of Health and Human Services, 2003). In addition, some state systems have developed staff hiring criteria and/or policies to ensure service providers possess specific skill sets (Frankel, Friedman, Johnson, Thies-Huber, & Zuiderveen, 2000).

Morrissey et al. (1997) and Backer (2000) found that beyond program characteristics, structural issues can greatly affect the success of a program, many of which are addressed through HFA state systems. These include the need for (a) community ownership and "buy-in," which entails engaging community members at all levels of the planning, implementation and evaluation processes; (b) sufficient and diverse funding to ensure program sustainability over long periods of time; (c) collaborative linkages across service organizations working towards a collective effort of community-wide prevention; and (d) media relations to raise awareness about the need for the program and indicate where services can be accessed.

Backer (2000) found that in addition to programmatic competence, capacity-building is necessary to sustain a prevention program. This includes organizational activities such as administration and management and technological capacities and resources. HFA state systems have evolved as a way to foster connections and stimulate ownership of the program. State systems tend to utilize the comprehensive skill sets (i.e., fundraising, advocacy, public, quality assurance, technology, media and community relations) of those involved with the program (state planners, funders, participants, volunteers, etc.) (PCA America, 2003b). This approach helps minimize the burden on program staff from having to be responsible for the wide-ranging and complex issues beyond providing program services and ensuring families get the support they need.

In their paper, *Resolving Paradoxes in the Expansion and Replication of Early Childhood Care and Education Programs*, Yoshikawa, Rosman, and Hsueh (2001) warn that replication should not be seen simply as the addition of programs. The authors state, "expansion and replication differ from simple aggregation (adding new sites) in that they involve higher levels of organization than program-level interaction" (p.17). They cite the example of Head Start, where the "replicating agency" itself contains many organizational levels including a training and technical assistance system and regional offices to support the growth of the program. The authors argue that replication must take into consideration both "horizontal relationships (e.g., interactions and support among programs), [and] vertical relationships (e.g., interaction between the replicating agency and individual program sites)" (p. 23). Within the vertical relationship, the intermediary organization has responsibilities to sites that typically include such activities as monitoring quality and providing technical assistance.

OUTCOMES OF A SYSTEMS APPROACH: FUNDING SUSTAINABILITY

Since sustainability is such a critical component of a program's survival, a natural question becomes: do state systems make a difference for the stability of a program? Using data from 34 states which responded to an annual state systems survey in 2002 (PCA America, 2003a), 17 states (50%) were categorized as more developed (i.e., having at least eight of the 10 centralized components mentioned earlier). Of these 17 well-developed state systems, 13 also responded to a Funding Survey which was conducted in 2003 (PCA America, 2003a). To assess the impact of state systems development on home visiting funding, information from both surveys was examined.

States with highly developed state systems had a larger number of HFA programs, with an average of 20 sites per state compared to five per state in states with less developed state systems ($p < .001$). Data from the annual 2001 HFA Site Profile (Harding, 2003) indicates that more developed states were serving an average of 2,186 families per state, compared to an average of 472 families in less developed states ($p < .01$).

Consistent with these figures, states with more developed systems reported larger budgets (M = 11.7 million) than those with less developed systems (M = 2.4 million), $p < .01$., and appeared to use a larger percentage of their budget to support state systems (averaging 16% vs. 4% in states with less developed systems, *ns*)[1]. *To some extent, these differences may be a factor of population size, as the 1999 population of children aged 0 to 5 years was somewhat larger in states with more developed state systems* ($p < .10$). It is also important to note that this finding is logical given that states with stronger systems tended to have a greater number of sites providing services to families.

How did these highly developed states fare with state budget cuts? This information is available only for 23 states responding to the Funding Survey, making differences difficult to discern. However, the percent of states maintaining their budget from 2002 to 2003 increased slightly along with the level of infrastructure development. Sixty-three percent of states who responded to the Funding Survey were able to maintain their budgets. Of these, more than one-half had a minimum of four components in place. This pattern of results suggests that having a well-developed state system provides noticeable benefits in terms of sustainability once states reach a certain level of development within a system (PCA America, 2003a). However, the fact that less developed states fared nearly as well suggests that there are a whole host of political, economic and social factors that contribute to the financial sustainability of a program. These findings certainly merit additional and more rigorous research to enable the field to discern if there are any causal relations between infrastructure and sustainability.

State Systems Benefits and Challenges

As cited in the *Framework for Healthy Families America State Systems Development* (PCA America, 2001) and recommended by researchers involved in program replication (Backer, 1991; Backer, 2000; Mihalic et al., 2004; Morrissey et al., 1997; Rogers, 1983; Rogers, 1995; Rogers & Kincaid, 1981), the inherent benefits and challenges to implementing and maintaining state systems are issues that continue to be discussed throughout the HFA network. State level planners embarking upon this process would be wise to engage all stakeholders and use a consensus building process that carefully considers how to maximize the benefits and address the challenges.

Benefits of State Systems

1. *Facilitate information sharing* by implementing and utilizing communication pathways. Many state systems have created vehicles for facilitating regular communication among sites throughout the state. These include maintaining a statewide listserv; convening regular meetings either in-person or via teleconference; hosting a website, chat room, or discussion boards; or disseminating a newsletter. The Every Child Succeeds program, which operates in Ohio and Kentucky, realized early on the need for effective two-way communication between the centralized management and decentralized service delivery system (see Ammerman, Putnam, Kopke, Gannon, Short, Van Ginkel et al., this volume).This communication is critical, particularly in states with rural sites that tend to be isolated and who benefit greatly by connecting with other sites (Backer, 1991; Mihalic et al., 2004; Morrissey et al., 1997; Nutbeam, 1996; PCA America, 2001; Rogers, 1995).

2. *Capitalize on state and local expertise.* Having a system in place creates opportunities for individuals who possess a range of expertise to be identified and utilized to provide supportive services to program staff and families (Mihalic et al., 2004; PCA America, 2001).
3. *Provide training and technical assistance.* Ongoing training and technical assistance to sites is a critical component of HFA. As new staff join programs and new programs develop, states with training and technical assistance systems ensure that sites can access training and technical assistance in a timely manner. As needs are identified by sites, the system responds to these needs either through developing new training programs or identifying experts in the community, state or region to provide wraparound trainings. A technical assistance system ensures that sites adhere to credentialing standards (Backer, 2000; Mihalic et al., 2004; Morrissey et al., 1997; PCA America, 2001).
4. *Advocate for programs* at the community and state levels through legislative activities, which contribute to long-term sustainability. States that have a system for advocacy monitor and react to pending legislation, provide training to site staff and families to enable them to advocate on the program's behalf, and cultivate relationships with key decisionmakers and political leaders (Morrissey et al., 1997; PCA America, 2001).
5. *Promote the value of high quality home visiting efforts.* States with marketing systems highlight the benefits of providing supportive services to parents. Resources dedicated to marketing and public relations enable a state to develop promotional materials, cultivate relationships with members of the press and seek out opportunities to increase awareness of HFA. State systems have been recognized by national institutions and Federal agencies which have been instrumental in bringing credibility to the program (Morrissey et al., 1997; PCA America, 2001; Strengthening America's Families, 1997; Thomas, Leicht, Hughes, Madigan, & Dowell, 2003).
6. *Identify and solicit funding.* There is no easy, systematic way to identify and secure multiple funding sources necessary for a system of assessment and home visitation services. To expect individual sites, that have a myriad of responsibilities, to monitor and apply for federal, state and local funds in addition to soliciting private and corporate dollars is a tall order. A system to identify appropriate sources of funding, prepare grant requests, monitor grant reporting

and perform certain fiduciary responsibilities is much more effective and efficient (Backer, 2000; Morrissey et al., 1997).

7. *Implement a statewide management information system* to monitor and evaluate services. Utilizing a common data management system, such as the Program Information Management System (PIMS) created by HFA, minimizes confusion, increases usability and meaningfulness of data for management at both the state and site levels, and simplifies staff workloads. It can also facilitate continuous quality improvement efforts to ensure model fidelity (see Ammerman et al., this volume). In addition, uniform definitions of data facilitate the comparison of findings from site to site (Harding, Reid, Oshana, Holton, & Representatives of the HFA Research Practice Council, 2004; Nutbeam, 1996; PCA America, 2001).

8. *Build consensus and partnerships*. An active state system can facilitate intra-agency collaboration with other state-level organizations. These partnerships reduce duplication of services and identify new training, technical assistance and fiscal resources. In addition, this type of collaboration provides opportunities for HFA systems to be incorporated into broader statewide efforts such as early childhood, child welfare and school readiness initiatives (Backer, 1991; PCA America, 2001, 2003b; Morrissey et al., 1997; Rogers, 1995).

9. *Create economies of scale*. A centralized system saves money. For instance, having in-state training eliminates the need to travel out-of-state or pay to have an outside trainer travel to multiple sites. It is also much more cost effective for a state to purchase a data management system (both hardware and software) used by sites than for each site to individually purchase their own unique system (PCA America, 2001).

10. *Facilitate the development of learning laboratories*. State systems encourage the cultivation of new ideas and approaches in which to support programs and families. This creativity results in the development of innovations (Nutbeam, 1996) such as distance learning which improve access to training throughout a state while minimizing costs associated with time away from the office. Healthy Families Florida, Healthy Families Indiana and Healthy Families Arizona have all incorporated feedback from sites to create a variety of distance learning modules (M. Pohutsky, personal communication, March 10, 2005; Schreiber & Friedman, 2004).

11. *Create a vision for the future.* When all sites are engaged in a strategic planning process for the state, individual sites are part of a larger whole. Sites contribute to a vision for the future of families in that state by developing a plan which identifies the goals, objectives, strategies and outcomes (Mihalic et al., 2004; PCA America, 2001).

Challenges of State Systems

Many of the challenges that may be encountered in the process of implementing a state system are similar to those encountered when establishing a coalition or collaborative partnership. Some challenges to consider include (PCA America, 2001):

Time. Having regular meetings, ensuring ongoing communication and working with system members to reach consensus on certain issues is undoubtedly time consuming. Many state leaders put in personal time above and beyond the requirements of their jobs. But the investment of time in building effective leadership and shared vision amongst key players in a state can pay off handsomely over the long haul (PCA America, 2001, 2003b).

System funding. In tight economic times, it is difficult to find resources to maintain the functions of a state system. Funders typically want to support direct service delivery, not "administrative functions." It is important to educate funders about the function of state systems and the centrality of that function to the quality and implementation of the program. State leaders responsible for funding must learn how to frame the interconnectedness of delivering quality services throughout a state and outcomes for families with young children (Backer, 2000; NCPCA, 1999; PCA America, 2001).

Turf issues. Organizations involved in various capacities related to different early childhood programs or who have a history with a single program may be competitive or resistant to collaboration, networking or sharing ideas for a statewide effort with a broader agenda. A state system helps unify such disparate agencies (Morrissey et al., 1997; PCA America, 2001).

The need to maintain a cadre of leaders who can support the system, particularly in times of transition. Leadership development is central to the ongoing operation of the state system. Programs must cultivate new leaders to assume statewide roles and ensure capacity. This leadership development is particularly important during times of program expansion (Mihalic et al., 2004; PCA America, 2001).

Maintaining a bond. In states where a program has grown incrementally over time, there tends to be a bond among individuals involved in the system. When a system changes and grows, some of the intimacy can be lost as a natural extension of that expansion. States should work to identify strategies to maintain connections between members of the system and archive the history of the system (Mihalic et al., 2004; PCA America, 2001; R. Ruffner & K. Whitaker, personal communication, October 8, 2004).

In spite of these challenges, the collective experience of the state leadership for HFA gathered through PCA America suggests that many states have thoughtfully and strategically addressed program implementation and promoted positive outcomes for children and families.

STATE EXAMPLES OF SYSTEMS DEVELOPMENT

Examples abound throughout the country of innovative practices at the system level. The following two case studies highlight particular developments in the areas of program expansion and evaluation.

State Systems and Program Expansion: Healthy Families Arizona

Arizona was one of the first states in the country to implement HFA. The program has been recognized as a noteworthy model by the Administration for Children and Families in their national scan of effective child abuse prevention programs (Thomas et al., 2003). Staff from Healthy Families Arizona (HFAz) has also assumed leadership of the Western Regional Resource Center.

Over the years of implementing HFAz, a strong bond formed between the multiple agencies providing a range of services to sites throughout the state (R. Ruffner & K. Whitaker, personal communication, October 8, 2004). These partners include the Department of Economic Security which administers funding contracts for the program. The department contracts with a private agency (LeCroy & Milligan Associates) to provide quality assurance training and technical assistance, develop a management information system and conduct ongoing evaluation (see Krysik & LeCroy, this volume, or http://www.healthyfamiliesarizona.org/ for more information.) Prevent Child Abuse Arizona (PCA Arizona), a chapter of PCA America, works closely with the program to provide advocacy support. All of these entities participate on both a statewide steering committee and a more extensive committee structure across the state. Due to the varied expertise on these committees, a feedback loop has been created that links outcome data from state evaluations to program practices. This loop creates a culture of constant self-exploration and innovation (R. Ruffner & K. Whitaker, personal communication, October 8, 2004) and helps to improve the "fit" between research and practice (Nutbeam, 1996; Perry, Murray, & Griffen, 1990).

Becky Ruffner of PCA Arizona and Kate Whitaker of LeCroy & Milligan believe that in spite of their various roles–everyone involved with HFAz is "pulling in the same direction" and is "unified in their purpose." This is precisely the type of shared vision found by Mihalic et al. (2004) to be critical for successful program implementation. HFAz has always considered its prevention work to be part of the continuum of child welfare services, and indeed a "prevention system" is the first recommendation of the state-level Child Protection Services Reform Commission (Prevention System Subcommittee of the Office of Arizona Governor Janet Napolitano, 2004). To that end, Governor Napolitano has stated that she intends to expand the program to all new parents who want services. The program's funding was doubled by the 2004 legislature, and the Governor's budget reflects an additional $5.5 million in the 2005 budget which will expand the number of sites statewide to nearly 50 (R. Ruffner & K. Whitaker, personal communication, October 8, 2004). This demonstrates the state's tremendous commitment towards the program as well as the capacity required to bring the program to scale.

> As Attorney General, I saw firsthand the impact of abuse and neglect on our children and the critical need for increased prevention efforts. As Arizona's twenty-first Governor, I have made it a priority to expand the Healthy Families Arizona program because it helps new parents succeed in keeping their children safe and healthy. Our state system–now serving over 100 local communities–is a model of excellence nationwide. –Arizona Governor Janet Napolitano

State Systems and Evaluation: Healthy Families Virginia

Data collected periodically by PCA America indicate that since the inception of HFA, more than 50% of states where the program exists have conducted some type of evaluation (Diaz et al., 2004; Harding, 2001; Schreiber & Friedman, 2004). In a few states, the evaluator is an integral part of the state system (PCA America, 2003b). Having this researcher-practitioner collaboration can be invaluable as it creates opportunities for two-way communication and allows for cross-disciplinary learning (Nutbeam, 1996). An example of this collaboration has occurred in

Virginia where evaluators from the College of William and Mary worked very closely with the program staff of Healthy Families Virginia (HFVa) to develop a comprehensive understanding of the program before any families were ever served. This university/community partnership facilitated mutual respect and learning between practitioners and researchers and enabled a valuable researcher-practitioner partnership to be established. Although the work of this initial group has long been completed, an evaluation subcommittee still regularly meets to discuss the needs of the sites across the state and plan a strategy for meeting new state requirements (J. Galano & L. Huntington, personal communication, August 4, 2003).

During the fiscal year 2002 legislative session, the funding for the program was not included in the Governor's budget. This meant that the program would have to fight for continued funding along with numerous other programs facing the same statewide crisis. HFVa received bi-partisan support and was the only program fully restored to the budget. The Executive Director of Prevent Child Abuse Virginia (PCA Virginia), the agency that coordinates the state system and who was involved with this process, felt that this success was due to two critical ingredients: persistent advocacy on the part of the sites and positive evaluation findings that clearly demonstrated that home visiting was a wise and necessary investment. Without the evaluation system in place, the program might have suffered a significant budget decrease (J. Schuchert, personal communication, April 12, 2002; PCA America, 2003b).

Lessons Learned from State Systems Development

In the seven years since the formalization of state systems, multiple opportunities to solicit feedback from members of the HFA network have enabled the authors to amass a great deal of systems implementation knowledge. This knowledge, accumulated via meetings, telephone and in-person conferences, is of particular interest to those individuals with state level planning responsibilities.

While anecdotal, these lessons learned represent the collective wisdom of those who have and continue to provide leadership around the development of state systems.

1. Be as inclusive as possible. Have representation from more than one home visiting group and the broader early childhood field. This representation can prove quite valuable for advocacy purposes, developing fundraising strategies and sharing resources. Efforts

to identify and recruit new partners should be ongoing and creative. Consider how to engage atypical messengers.

2. Develop a thoughtful strategic plan and refer to it often. This document, used properly, should lay the foundation of the state system and be referred to as a guide for all major activities. It can be utilized for a variety of purposes such as delineating roles and responsibilities of members of the system, establishing a benchmark in which to measure progress, aligning members of the system on the mission and goals, and for advocacy, fundraising, training, partnerships and promotional purposes.

3. Facilitate opportunities to have members of the network from all levels meet on a regular basis. This fosters team-building and keeping members of the system abreast of policy and procedure changes, and provides opportunities to network, identify resources and resolve issues that could have a statewide impact. Honor and celebrate successes.

4. Develop advocacy training for advisory committees, staff and families to empower them to advocate for services that are important to them. Ensure that there is a ready cadre of people who can speak to policymakers from their own experiences at a lobbying day or legislative hearing. A state chapter of Voices for America's Children or local grassroots groups can be helpful in this work.

5. Whenever possible, seek out opportunities to provide positive media coverage of the program and system. This is an important step in increasing awareness among the public and key policymakers. Provide media training for staff and families so they are prepared in the event the program or state has an opportunity to obtain some publicity. Contact a local community college that has a communications department to help identify potential resources to provide this training.

6. Advocate for funding to support the state systems infrastructure. Secure funding for a statewide coordinator who can help ensure that basic functions such as training and technical assistance are met.

7. Have a commitment to building quality local programs, efficient state systems and evaluation which informs training and practice simultaneously and in an integrated way.

8. Be patient. Building systems is painstaking work that takes a lot of time. Although convening entities from around the state and getting them to agree on priorities and strategies can be a frustrating process, it provides the chance to build leadership which will lead to better results in the end.

CONCLUSION

As research justifies the importance of creating and maintaining state systems, the experiences and history of the HFA initiative are further validated. State systems facilitate the leveraging of funds, ensure high quality replication of programs and provide opportunities for leadership development. Put simply, systems increase program capacity to deliver services to families. State systems and Regional Resource Centers will help ensure that HFA will exist long into the future, regardless of the challenges that may arise. The lessons learned from the HFA experience can be applied to multiple social service and family support programs, well outside of the realm of home visitation. The key components of systems-building efforts are universal to any type of thoughtful and responsible program development. Success in this area bodes well for the long-term development and sustainability of direct service programs.

More research is needed to describe and demonstrate the impact and reach of systems work. Particularly, research needs to find new ways of evaluating systems so that a range of outcomes can adequately assess the process and impact of system-building. The better the impact of system-building can be demonstrated, the more likely funders will see the value in investing in critical infrastructure to support growing programs.

NOTE

1. Only three of the less-developed states reported the percentage of their budget used to support a state system, making this comparison difficult to test statistically. Other data suggest that many of the less-developed state systems do not have official funding for state functions, but rather operate through in-kind contributions of coalition members or site representatives sharing their expertise with others in their state.

REFERENCES

Ammerman, R., Putnam, F., Kopke, J., Gannon, T., Short, J., Van Ginkel, J. et al. (in press). Development and implementation of a quality assurance infrastructure in a multisite home visitation program in Ohio and Kentucky. *Journal of Prevention & Intervention in the Community.*

Backer, T. E. (1991). *Dissemination and utilization strategies for foundations: Adding value to grantmaking.* Kansas City, MO: Ewing M. Kauffman Foundation.

Backer, T. E. (1995). Reviewing the behavioral science knowledge base on technology transfer. *NIDA Research Monograph, 155.*

Backer, T. E. (2000). The failure of success: Challenges of disseminating effective substance abuse prevention programs. *Journal of Community Psychology, 28,* 353-373.

Bruner, C. (1996). *Steps along an uncertain path: State initiatives promoting comprehensive, community-based reform.* Washington, DC: Center for the Study of Social Policy.

Diaz, J., Oshana, D., & Harding, K. (2004). *Healthy Families America 2003 profile of program sites.* Chicago: Prevent Child Abuse America.

Frankel, S., Friedman, L., Johnson, A., Thies-Huber, A., & Zuiderveen, S. (2000). *Healthy Families America: Site development guide.* Chicago: Prevent Child Abuse America.

Green, L. W. (2001). From research to "best practices" in other setting and populations. *American Journal of Health Behavior, 25,* 165-178.

Harding, K. (2003). *Healthy Families America annual site profile report.* Chicago: Prevent Child Abuse America.

Harding, K., Reid, R., Oshana, D., Holton, J., & Representatives of the Healthy Families America Research Council (2004). *Initial results of the HFA Implementation Study. A report submitted to the David and Lucille Packard Foundation.* Chicago: Prevent Child Abuse America.

Harding, K., Galano, J., Huntington, L., Martin, J., & Schellenbach, C. (in press). HFA effectiveness: A synthesis of support. *Journal of Prevention & Intervention in the Community.*

Innovative Strategies: *Staff retention* (n.d.). Retrieved July 15, 2005, from http://www.healthyfamiliesamerica.org/network_resources/is_staff_retention.shtml

Krysik, J., & LeCroy, L. (in press). The evaluation of Healthy Families Arizona: A multisite home visitation program. *Journal of Prevention & Intervention in the Community.*

Mihalic, S., Irwin, K., Fagan, A., Ballard, D., & Elliott, D. (2004, July). *Successful program implementation: Lessons from blueprints.* Juvenile Justice Bulletin. Retrieved July 12, 2005, from http://www.ncjrs.org/pdffiles1/ojjdp/204273.pdf

Morrissey, E., Wandersman, A., Seybolt, D., Nation, M., Crusto, C., & Davino, K. (1997). Toward a framework for bridging the gap between science and practice in prevention: A focus on evaluator and practitioner perspectives. *Evaluation and Program Planning, 20,* 367-377.

National Committee to Prevent Child Abuse (1995). *Healthy Families America third year progress report.* Chicago: Author.

National Committee to Prevent Child Abuse (1997). *Healthy Families America: Five years of building stronger families.* Chicago: Author.

National Committee to Prevent Child Abuse (1999). *Proceedings from the State Leaders meeting.* Chicago: Author.

Nutbeam, P. (1996). Achieving 'best practice' in health promotion: Improving the fit between research and practice. *Health Education Research, 11,* 317-326.

Perry, C. L., Murray, D. M., & Griffen, G. (1990). Evaluating statewide dissemination of smoking prevention curricula: Factors in teacher compliance. *Journal of School Health, 60,* 501-504.

Prevent Child Abuse America (2001). *Framework for Healthy Families America state systems development.* Chicago: Author.

Prevent Child Abuse America (2003a). *Home visiting legislation and funding: Lessons from Healthy Families America.* Chicago: Author.

Prevent Child Abuse America (2003b). *State systems development guide.* Chicago: Author.

Prevent Child Abuse America (2004a). *Healthy Families America credentialing manual.* Chicago: Author.

Prevent Child Abuse America (2004b). *Healthy Families America peer reviewer manual.* Chicago: Author.

Prevention System Subcommittee of the Office of Arizona Governor Janet Napolitano (2004, September). *Action plan for reform of Arizona's child protection system.* Retrieved July 13, 2005, from http://www.governor.state.az.us/cps/documents/NeglectPreventionSystem-Gov%27sOfficeFinal.pdf

Rogers, E. M. (1983). *Diffusion of innovations.* New York: Free Press; London: Collier Macmillan.

Rogers, E. M. (1995). *Diffusion of innovations.* New York: Free Press.

Rogers, E. M., & Kincaid, D. L. (1981). *Communication networks: Toward a new paradigm for research.* New York: Free Press.

Salus, M. K. (2004). *Supervising child protective services caseworkers.* Washington, DC: U.S. Department of Health and Human Services, Administration for Children and Families. Retrieved July 26, 2005 from http://nccanch.acf.hhs.gov/pubs/usermanuals/supercps/ supercps.pdf

Schorr, L. B. (1997). *Common purpose: Strengthening families and communities to rebuild America.* New York: Anchor Books.

Schreiber, L., & Friedman, L. (2004). *State of state systems in 2004.* Unpublished raw data.

Strengthening America's Families. *Effective family programs for prevention of delinquency.* Retrieved June 22, 2005 from http://www.strengtheningfamilies.org/html/model_programs.html

Thomas, D., Leicht, C., Hughes, C., Madigan, A., & Dowell, K. (2003). *Emerging practices in the prevention of child abuse and neglect.* Washington, DC: Office on Child Abuse and Neglect, Department of Health and Human Services.

U.S. Department of Health and Human Services (2003). *Child welfare: HHS could play a greater role in helping child welfare agencies recruit and retain staff.* (GAO-03-357). Washington, DC: Author.

Weissberg, R. P., Gullotta, T. P., Hampton, R. L., Ryan, B. A., & Adams, G. R. (1997). *Dissemination of prevention programs, establishing preventive services.* London: Sage Publications.

Yoshikawa, H., Rosman, E. A., & Hsueh, J. (2001). *Resolving paradoxes in the expansion and replication of early childhood care and education programs.* New York: New York University.

doi:10.1300/J005v34n01_04

APPENDIX A

WHAT IS QUALITY FOR HEALTHY FAMILIES AMERICA?
THE HEALTHY FAMILIES AMERICA CREDENTIALING SYSTEM

The purpose of credentialing is to ensure that any entity utilizing the Healthy Families America (HFA) name represents an abiding commitment to deliver the highest quality services possible to families and children. The development of the credentialing system was initiated as a result of discussions among members of the HFA network in the early days of the initiative. At issue was how to best assure quality once the excitement of planning a program and training staff began to fade and the day-to-day realities of operating a program–and the attendant pressures to dilute its quality–began to mount. PCA America's Board of Directors decided that HFA should proceed with the development of a credentialing system to maintain its quality.

One of the primary challenges to the development of credentialing was determining how to promote flexibility while ensuring that quality standards were being met. This balance was accomplished by identifying the core concepts upon which common programmatic practice was based. These core concepts are known as the *critical elements*. Defined by more than 20 years of research, these elements represent a compilation of knowledge about how best to serve overburdened families (PCA America, 2004a, 2004b).

While pilot test results showed that the basic process worked well for individual programs with simple administrative structures, such was not the case with large, multi-site state systems because the functions of the central administration were not fully measured. As a result, PCA America, with the generous support of the Pritzker Cousins Foundation, expanded the credentialing process to assess quality in HFA multi-site state systems (PCA America, 2004a).

As of publication, over 68% of the HFA sites have successfully gone through the credentialing process and four states have attained the multi-site credential, with more in process (C. Wessel, personal communication, June 8, 2006).

Development and Implementation
of a Quality Assurance Infrastructure
in a Multisite Home Visitation Program
in Ohio and Kentucky

Robert T. Ammerman

Cincinnati Children's Hospital Medical Center

Frank W. Putnam

*Cincinnati Children's Hospital Medical Center
and University of Cincinnati College of Medicine*

Jonathan E. Kopke

Institute for the Study of Health, University of Cincinnati

Thomas A. Gannon
Jodie A. Short
Judith B. Van Ginkel
Margaret J. Clark

*Cincinnati Children's Hospital Medical Center
and University of Cincinnati College of Medicine*

Mark A. Carrozza

Institute for Policy Research, University of Cincinnati

Alan R. Spector

Quality Assurance Consultant, Private Consultant

Address correspondence to: Robert T. Ammerman, PhD, Cincinnati Children's Hospital Medical Center, 3333 Burnet Avenue, Cincinnati, OH 45229 (E-mail: robert. ammerman@cchmc.org).

[Haworth co-indexing entry note]: "Development and Implementation of a Quality Assurance Infrastructure in a Multisite Home Visitation Program in Ohio and Kentucky." Ammerman, Robert T. et al. Co-published simultaneously in *Journal of Prevention & Intervention in the Community* (The Haworth Press, Inc.) Vol. 34, No.1/2, 2007, pp. 89-107; and: *The Healthy Families America® Initiative: Integrating Research, Theory and Practice* (ed: Joseph Galano) The Haworth Press, Inc., 2007, pp. 89-107. Single or multiple copies of this article are available for a fee from The Haworth Document Delivery Service [1-800-HAWORTH, 9:00 a.m. - 5:00 p.m. (EST). E-mail address: docdelivery@haworthpress.com].

SUMMARY. As home visitation programs go to scale, numerous challenges are faced in implementation and quality assurance. This article describes the origins and implementation of Every Child Succeeds, a multisite home visitation program in southwestern Ohio and Northern Kentucky. In order to optimize quality assurance and generate new learning for the field, a Web-based system (eECS) was designed to systematically collect and use data. Continuous quality assurance procedures derived from business and industry have been established. Findings from data collection have documented outcomes, and have identified clinical needs that potentially undermine the impact of home visitation. An augmented module approach has been used to address these needs, and a program to treat maternal depression is described as an example of this approach. Challenges encountered are also discussed.
doi:10.1300/J005v34n01_05 *[Article copies available for a fee from The Haworth Document Delivery Service: 1-800-HAWORTH. E-mail address: <docdelivery@haworthpress.com> Website: <http://www.HaworthPress.com>*
© 2007 by The Haworth Press, Inc. All rights reserved.]

KEYWORDS. Home visitation, child abuse prevention, quality assurance

INTRODUCTION

Home visitation is a prevention strategy whereby trained professionals or paraprofessionals deliver services to young mothers and their children. Initially designed to prevent child abuse and neglect, home visitation has expanded its focus to provide a range of supports and services to optimize the development of young children. As noted by Gomby (1999), home visitation programs have proliferated in the United States. Fueled by encouraging findings from several key studies (see Karoly et al., 1998), many localities and regions have embraced home visitation as an approach to preventing child abuse and neglect. Although there is a vigorous debate about the most effective approach to home visiting (Leventhal, 2005), there is widespread commitment to home visitation as a core feature of early prevention (Guterman, 2001).

It is useful to collect the experiences of programs that emerge from and are embedded in the community. For example, Galano et al. (2001) described the social and political processes that led to the development and growth of the Hampton Healthy Family Partnership in Virginia. Strategies for navigating and accommodating the multiple interests and influences were articulated, and serve as a helpful guide to establishing prevention programs on a large scale (Racine, 1998). Moreover, with increasing emphasis on accountability and documenting outcomes in prevention programs, it is essential to conduct ongoing evaluations. Evaluation can be used to improve services and facilitate the evolution of programs towards increased effectiveness, and to measure and document changes over time.

This article describes Every Child Succeeds (ECS), a home visitation program for first-time, at-risk mothers in southwestern Ohio and northern Kentucky. Specifically, four areas are addressed. First, we recount the origins of ECS, with particular attention to constituencies that identified the need, garnered the resources for prevention services, selected the approach and designed the program's configuration. Second, we describe the infrastructure for the gathering, management, and use of data, which is a core feature of the ECS Model (comprising our approach to organizing and delivering home visitation services). The processes by which this infrastructure was designed and implemented are covered in considerable detail, as we believe that such a system is indispensable to maximize the potential of home visiting programs to yield high quality data for evaluation and quality improvement purposes. Moreover, we believe that prevention programs will increasingly be called upon to develop similar evaluation and program operation data systems, and that the sharing of our experiences is of value to the field. Third, we describe Continuous Quality Improvement (CQI) and program accountability procedures, present selected outcomes, and review an augmented module approach to enriching home visitation that grew out of learning derived from evaluation findings. Finally, challenges and impediments are reviewed.

EVERY CHILD SUCCEEDS

Program Overview

ECS is a large-scale, community-based home visitation program for first-time mothers and their children. Administered by Cincinnati Children's Hospital Medical Center, ECS utilizes two national models of home visitation–Healthy Families America® (HFA; Daro & Harding, 1999) and Nurse-Family Partnership (NFP; Olds, Hill, O'Brien, Racine, & Moritz, 2004). Eligible mothers are at-risk for adverse parenting outcomes, as reflected by at least one of four targeted risk characteristics: unmarried; inadequate income (up to 300% of poverty level, Medicaid, reported concerns about finances); under 18 years of age; and late, no, or inadequate prenatal care. Mothers are enrolled prenatally (HFA and NFP) through the child reaching 3 months of age (HFA only), and regular home visits are provided (depending on the model) by trained nurses, social workers, or related professionals and paraprofessionals. Home visits are provided until the child reaches age 2 (NFP) or 3 (HFA), starting intensively and tapering over time. The goals of ECS are to (a) improve pregnancy outcomes through nutrition education and substance use reduction; (b) support parents in providing children with a safe, nurturing, and stimulating home environment; (c) optimize child health and development; (d) link families to health care and other needed services; and (e) promote economic self-sufficiency.

ECS oversees a collaborative of 15 contracted agencies, which provide home visitation in seven counties in southwestern Ohio and northern Kentucky. Since its founding in 1999, ECS has provided over 210,000 home visits to 10,000 families. Demographic and risk characteristics of mothers are presented in Table 1. It is noteworthy that a high proportion of mothers exhibit clinical features that have been implicated in maladaptive parenting, including elevated levels of depression (44%) and histories of

TABLE 1. *Demographic and risk characteristics of ECS mothers.* All data collected at enrollment for all mothers with the exception of depression data which were derived from a subsample (N = 806; Ammerman, Putnam, Altaye et al., 2005).

Mean age:	20.5 years (SD = 4.6)
Race:	
Caucasian:	64%
African American:	33%
Other:	3%
Unmarried:	85%
18 years or younger:	35%
Low Income:	78%
Inadequate prenatal care:	24%
Socially isolated:	75%
Multiple stressors:	78%
Depressed in 1st year of service:	44%
Trauma history	69%

interpersonal trauma (69%, such as child abuse, sexual abuse, and witnessing violence). In addition, we estimate that about 50% of ECS participants are Appalachian, a group that is at risk for a variety of social problems (e.g., early school dropout, unemployment).

EVALUATION AND INFORMATION MANAGEMENT

Compelling Need for Information Management Infrastructure

It was rapidly apparent that the centralized management and decentralized service delivery system required smooth and efficient two-way communication to work effectively. The central administration required standardized, high-quality data on service parameters to inform its allocation of resources, coordination of multiple funding streams, program consistency, quality assurance, and outcome evaluation. Provider agencies, with their local knowledge and community concerns, required clear direction and policy support from the administration as they sought to implement and, to some extent, adapt program models to their resources and agency culture. With over 120 home visitors, agency supervisors, and support staff in the field, clear and consistent communication was essential to managing a high-quality, standardized program that could be uniformly evaluated across multiple provider sites. In addition, another set of stakeholders including funders, community supporters, politicians, the media, and the community at large were requesting information on the scope and impacts of the program. Although the aforementioned needs are typical of multisite prevention programs, we found little guidance in the literature about how to construct an information management system that maximized efficiency and served multiple purposes.

Origins of the Web-Based System

ECS first utilized a paper-based information management system. The inadequacy of the paper-based system, particularly for a large-scale prevention program, led to consideration of alternative information management systems. Several pre-packaged software systems were examined and ultimately rejected because they were overly generic and relatively inflexible. We elected to develop a new Web-based system, and enlisted the participation of home visitors, supervisors, and administrators, in addition to evaluation staff and Web designers. This group identified issues to be addressed and features that would be essential to a Web-based system, including the following:

1. Collection of service provision data and documentation of services provided and billed.
2. Maintenance of family service or case records, including demographics, scores on screening and evaluation measures that dictated types and levels of service, and related information.
3. Collection of eligibility information for multiple payment streams, which vary by state and county.
4. Documentation of fulfillment of state requirements, such as timely completion of Individualized Family Service Plans (IFSPs).
5. Rapid collection and analysis of quality assurance benchmarks for management and clinical supervision at both the agency and home visitor levels.
6. Simplification and standardization of billing procedures to reduce the enormous paperwork involved in submitting and verifying billing.
7. Large, multisite, aggregated datasets for strategic planning and long-term resource allocations.
8. Common communication forum in which ECS management could post system-wide information on policy changes, training opportunities, and general announcements.
9. Ability of each agency to retrieve its own data for supervision and quality control.
10. Ability to quickly query system-wide or regional data to respond to outside questions and requests.
11. Ability to have a "real-time" monitoring of service demands so that monthly visit quotas could be equitably distributed among multiple sites and reallocated efficiently as needed to ensure full utilization of time-limited monies.
12. Ability to collect standardized evaluation data for research studies embedded within the larger service delivery system.
13. The need to interface with multiple other data systems (e.g., Medicaid, Ohio and Kentucky early intervention services).

Design and Development Strategy

Creating a Web-based system is a daunting task. Indeed, in a review of computer implementation projects in business and industry, The Standish Group (1995) determined that, in companies comparable in size to ECS, only 28% of computer projects were "completely successful," and at least 31% of all computer projects were eventually abandoned because they were "hopelessly unsuccessful." Even among projects that were not abandoned, at least 25% ultimately delivered fewer than half of their originally planned features. While competent software developers are essential to the success of any computer project, the authors noted that the developers' influence on a project's final outcome was typically dwarfed by other factors including: (a) degree of end-user involvement, (b) level of executive management support, and (c) clarity and focus of the project definition.

Consequently, as ECS developed a customized Web-based data system, we strived to include home visitors, supervisors, and administrators in all aspects of the process (Kopke et al., 2003). Through regular meetings, prototypes of data collection forms, procedures for uploading data and accessing summary reports, and the "look and feel" of the Web-based system were reviewed with agency representatives. Such a process engaged the enthusiasm and support of collaborative partners, and increased the likelihood that the final product would be effective, efficient, and usable.

The interrelationships among the various forms and measures were carefully scrutinized at this stage with particular attention being paid to maintaining "referential integrity" (e.g., each Home Visit Form must be associated with one and only one mother's account to avoid "orphaned" records), and "third normal form" (e.g., the database logs each infant birth date only once, even though that date must be collected on two different forms). Maintaining third normal form not only minimizes the size of the database, but also ensures that the database is internally consistent. Although primarily technical concerns, these issues resulted in changes to data collection procedures in the field and underscore the importance of a synergistic collaboration between service providers and software developers.

Designing the Web Site

Design of eECS was influenced by Krug's (2000) book entitled *Don't Make Me Think,* a guide to constructing intuitive and "user friendly" Web sites. Krug approaches Web design from what he calls the Trunk Test Of Usability: "Imagine that you've been blindfolded and locked in the trunk of a car, then driven around for a while and dumped on a page somewhere deep in the bowels of a Web site. If the page is well designed, you should be able to answer these questions without hesitation: What site is this? What page am I on? What are the major sections of this site? What are my options at this level?" (p. 87).

As shown in a sample screen shot from eECS (Figure 1), the influence of Krug and other Web design experts led us to incorporate the following usability augmenters into the design of our online data system: (a) Each page incorporates "persistent navigation elements"–clickable graphics that appear in identical positions on every page to represent the major sections of the system, and to indicate the user's current location within the system. (b) Although the Help button is a persistent navigation element that appears identically on every page, it is "context sensitive" in that clicking it always invokes a Help screen that is tailored to the current page. (c) The heading of every Web page includes a series of clickable links that allow users to directly return to any pages they passed through on their way from the home page to the current page. (d) We rely on conventional page elements that are familiar to Internet users, such as round "radio buttons"

FIGURE 1. A sample eECS Web page showing a typical data form. Features of the design that optimize usability and efficiency include the persistent navigation elements, ways to reverse mistakes, links to move through the system, and conventional page elements.

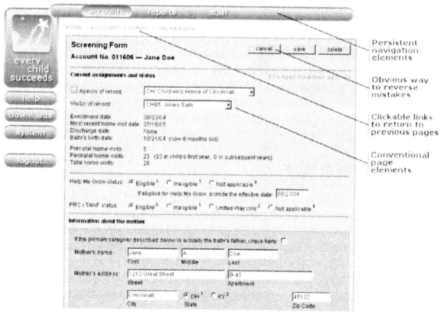

Source: Every Child Succeeds. Used with Permission.

and square checkboxes. (e) At every point in the system, we provide an obvious way for users to un-do what they have just done. Users who do not see an obvious way out of a mistake will often become frustrated and re-sort to risky responses, such as turning off their computers. Therefore, we always provide a recognizable way to back out of any page that was erroneously entered, or delete any record that was inadvertently saved. (f) Wherever possible, Web pages perform validity checks on each field before submitting values to the server. For example, entering the incorrect date of February 30 triggers an error message while the mistake can still be corrected at its point of origin. (g) We designed our Web site for "complexity hiding." That is, users with lower levels of access authority can see no indication that the Web site includes features beyond those that are open to them. In fact, more than half the features of the system are completely hidden from everyone except the few persons with the top-ranking System Administrator role. (h) Wherever possible, we avoided free-form text fields. Multiple-choice questions are far quicker for data-entry purposes, and they are far less ambiguous. The sample Web page (shown in Figure 1) also demonstrates the integration of information that is helpful to the home visitor (e.g., number of visits, date of most recent visit) and financial administrators (e.g., funder eligibility). Combining such information increases efficiency and eliminates artificial barriers between program functions.

PRODUCTS AND OUTCOMES: EVALUATION, CONTINUOUS QUALITY IMPROVEMENT, AND AUGMENTED MODULES

Evaluation and Outcomes

Development of the ECS evaluation was guided by three principles. First, an ongoing evaluation is integral to quality service. Evaluations of social service programs are often viewed as secondary efforts that are separate and distinct from the intervention, which in part contributes to the perception among many providers that evaluations are burdensome and detract from the primary objective of providing services. The ECS evaluation is integrated with home visitation through the use of measures that, in addition to providing important information regarding outcomes and related issues, enhance the quality of service. For example, screening for maternal depression not only yields information about the prevalence of depression, but also alerts home visitors to the need for mental health treatment and to adapt home visitation to meet the unique challenges associated with maternal depression. Integration is also achieved by weaving the timing of administration of measures into the ongoing service, such as using a measure of smoking and substance use administered prior to talking with mothers about the negative health consequences of substance use, dangers of secondhand smoke, etc. Second, the evaluation addresses areas important to the multiple stakeholders and consumers of home visitation programs, including funders, legislators, policymakers, clients, and the communities served by the program. Third, the evaluation yields data that guide improvement efforts and facilitate the evolution of home visitation towards increased efficiency and effectiveness.

The ECS evaluation consists of selected measures administered multiple times over the course of home visitation. There is a concentration of measures at the start and end of home visitation; measures are given intermittently over the course of service so as not to cluster too many at any given interval. Measures consist of maternal self-report, maternal report documented by home visitors, and home visitor observation. Using a mixture of standardized and unstandardized measures, domains measured include child developmental status, home environment, maternal mental health, maternal substance use, maternal trauma history, parenting attitudes, social support, and maternal life course. Domains are categorized as being outcomes (e.g., child developmental status), potential moderators of outcomes (e.g., trauma history), or process (e.g., frequency of home visits). Home visitors receive training in administration of measures, and are provided with ongoing technical assistance. Additional program trainings that cover domains measured in the evaluation (e.g., trauma survivors) also include reviews of the corresponding instrument. The evaluation design is quasi-experimental, in that all mothers participate in home visitation. Outcomes are compared to benchmarked objectives in order to document results. Benchmarks are determined by published findings from similar samples where available. Also, pre-post (and midpoint) comparisons on measures are used to monitor changes over time. We have particularly focused attention on variables that can impact home visitation (e.g., maternal depression, social support), which in turn has led to an augmented modules approach to enrich the program (see below). Table 2 shows representative outcomes derived from the evaluation of ECS.

Continuous Quality Improvement and Program Accountability

Primary concepts of Continuous Quality Improvement (CQI) and program accountability emerged from business and manufacturing (Deming,

TABLE 2. Representative Outcomes of Mothers and Children in Every Child Succeeds

---

- *Child's source of medical care.* At one year, 94% of children are receiving regular and consistent medical care from a documented pediatric practice or clinic.
- *Infant mortality.* During child's first year, mortality rate is 60% lower (Donovan et al., 2007).
- *Child development.* At end of service, 88% of children have no delays (Denver Developmental Screening Test-II; Frankenburg et al., 1996) in Language, 93% in Personal Development, 93% in Fine Motor, and 94% in Gross Motor.
- *Parenting attitudes and beliefs.* At end of service, mothers report beliefs and attitudes (Adult-Adolescent Parenting Inventory; Bavolek & Keene, 1999) consistent with nurturing and effective parenting (99%), meeting the emotional needs of their children (93%). and having realistic expectations for behavior and development (87%).
- *Stimulating and nurturing home environment.* At end of service, home environments (HOME Inventory; Caldwell & Bradley, 1984) contain stimulating learning materials (98%), are conducive to learning (97%), and have high maternal involvement (97%).
- *Maternal depression.* 51% with elevated levels of depression (using Beck Depression Inventory-II; Beck, Steer, & Brown, 1996) at enrollment are not depressed at 9 months.
- *Maternal employment and education.* 86% are employed and/or in school during their participation in ECS.
- *Referral to community resources.* Over the course of service, 69% of mothers and children are linked to other resources in their communities, including housing, day care, medical care, and domestic violence shelters.
- *Consumer satisfaction.* At the end of service, 99% of mothers report overall satisfaction with the program.

1982; Juran, 1992). Specifically, CQI is a systematic approach to improving processes and outcomes through regular data collection, examination of performance relative to predetermined targets, review of practices that promote or impede improvement, and application of changes in practices that may lead to improvements in performance. The foundation of CQI is the collection and regular use of data in an ongoing fashion. Through regular monitoring, organizations can identify and rectify impediments to effective performance, and document changes and improvements.

Although CQI is a relatively standard practice in business, it has been adopted slowly by other fields (Bickman & Noser, 1999). CQI methods have been applied to health care, with documented improvements in care quality (Solberg, Brekke, Kottke, & Steel, 1998). With only a few exceptions (Domitrovich & Greenberg, 2000), CQI methods have not been widely used in the prevention field. In addition, despite several recommendations that CQI methods be used in home visitation programs (e.g., Olds, 2003; Thompson, Kropenske, Heinicke, Gomby, & Halfon, 2001), there are few published reports on their use. Yet, there are compelling reasons for home visitation programs to adopt CQI procedures. For example, home visitation programs particularly those operating on a large scals, often have difficulty maintaining model fidelity in the face of idiosyncratic local and regional influences that disrupt or interfere with optimal implementation. Adapting home visitation models to the unique community settings in which they reside is best accomplished through CQI methods, which allow organizations and individual sites to focus on problems that may be unique to them. In addition, CQI methods provide a means for community-based programs to benchmark their processes and outcomes, thereby documenting results in the absence of control or comparison groups that may be unavailable or infeasible.

The CQI and program accountability methods used by ECS emphasize providing home visitors and agencies with regular reports summarizing their performances on a variety of quality indicators reflecting processes and outcomes. Most of these reports are directly obtainable by agencies through eECS. For each agency and for ECS as a whole, performance is gauged against (a) preestablished targets, (b) performance of other agencies, and (c) averages across agencies. A CQI Team, which is composed of agency, administration, and evaluation representatives, meets regularly to review quality indicator targets and assess agency and system-wide performance. This entity also establishes targets based on program standards, funder requirements, and goals of the program.

The most important CQI report is the Red/Green Chart. Adapted from manufacturing and other business models, the Red/Green Chart displays performance on quality indicators as having met or exceeded preestablished targets (colored in green) or as falling short of targets (colored in red). Examination of the Red/Green Chart immediately yields specific areas of strength or weakness for a particular agency, patterns of performance for an agency as a whole, and patterns of performance for a specific quality indicator across agencies. Specific areas of weakness in an agency are addressed in Agency Action Plans, which are prepared and reviewed quarterly with the input of the agency. Targeted areas of improvement are identified in Agency Action Plans, and procedures to bring about improvement are delineated based upon individual agency needs and learned practices from more effective agencies. Extensive underperformance may require major system changes, whereas more circumscribed areas of weakness may be rectified with relatively minor procedural changes or additional training and support. Quality indicators that are "red" across multiple agencies may reflect an overly ambitious performance target, or a pervasive shortcoming in practice. Quality indicators that are consistently "green" across agencies necessitate an increase in the target in order to promote continued improvement. These charts are regularly reviewed by the CQI Team. In addition to the Red/Green Chart, reports are regularly available to agencies regarding individual home visitor performance, outcomes achieved by home visitors and agencies, and clinical activities of home visitors. A Change Management Committee convenes to approve system changes, thereby discouraging the adoption of idiosyncratic, agency-specific procedural changes that may increase interagency variability and decrease quality. This combination of regular reports, their direct accessibility by agencies, and a system for reviewing performance and implementing strategies to ensure continued quality, is the foundation of CQI and performance accountability.

Because CQI is driven by performance data, a prerequisite for its success is the degree to which agencies seek information about their performance. Through eECS, a count of the number of times that agencies download reports is available, thereby providing an index of use of performance data. Since the inception of the report access feature, in contrast to the limited numbers of centrally prepared reports available to agencies prior to eECS, there has been an increase of 297% in the number of reports obtained by agencies. Agencies access reports at a high rate, and there has been a consistent increase in report downloading over time, indicating an increased interest in obtaining performance information. Figure 2 shows the effects of CQI strategies on the improvement of specific performance indicators by an agency. It displays the proportion of prenatal enrollments for HFA Agency A and the number of reports of this information accessed by the agency (ECS has an initiative to increase the proportion of prenatal referrals) during a five-quarter period. At the start, Agency A was below the target proportion of 65%. The agency examined its procedures for enrolling mothers prenatally, and implemented changes designed to increase prenatal enrollment rates. The graph shows the percentage of newly enrolled mothers (right y-axis) who were recruited prenatally and the total number of performance reports accessed (left y-axis) by Agency A. Results indicate a steady increase to the ECS target of 65% of referrals done prenatally, an increase likely brought about by changes in the procedures used by Agency A to identify and enroll new mothers during pregnancy. There was also a parallel rise in the number of reports accessed, reflecting the agency's use of data to monitor prenatal enrollment rates over time and observe the impact of changes in recruitment procedures.

Note that, in the above CQI procedure, it is not possible to definitively establish a causal connection between implementing a change plan, accessing reports, and subsequent improvements in indicators. Meeting such a standard is neither necessary nor feasible in the context of a community-based prevention program, and it is not part of CQI efforts in business and industry. Rather, the repeated demonstration of improvements

FIGURE 2. Number of reports accessed and corresponding increase in proportion of prenatal enrollments over five quarters for Agency A

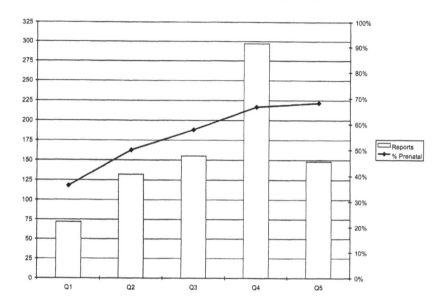

using these procedures in an iterative way, provides support for the use of CQI as a means to enhance home visitation.

Enriching Home Visitation Through Augmented Modules

Home visitation programs are based on the assumption that at-risk mothers and their children will benefit from education, training, and support. Yet, as home visitation has matured, it has become evident that there are barriers to families optimally benefiting from the service. These include maternal mental health problems, substance abuse, and domestic violence. In order to maximize the effectiveness of home visitation, these barriers need to be addressed. However, there is little guidance from the empirical literature on how to adapt home visitation to meet the needs of families compromised by significant clinical and social problems. At ECS, we have elected to address these issues through augmenting standard home visitation services with additional interventions, or augmented modules. In order to be fully beneficial, we believe that modules must: (a) meet a need that is not explicitly addressed in home visitation; (b) address issues that are important to family well-being and may adversely impact home visitation; (c) support home visitors who may not be adequately prepared to address a particular need (LeCroy & Whitaker, 2005); and (d) work closely with home visitation services to promote collaboration, mutually benefit both home visitation and the targeted need of the module, and minimze overlap in efforts.

The Maternal Depression Module (MDM) is an example of an augmented module. The MDM provides treatment to depressed mothers participating in home visitation, and was developed for four reasons. First, measurement of maternal depression in ECS revealed a high prevalence rate. In a sample of 806 mothers enrolled in ECS, 44% had elevated levels of depression (14 or higher on the Beck Depression Inventory-II) during the first nine months (based on measurements at enrollment and nine months later) of service (Ammerman, Putnam, Altaye et al., 2007). Second, despite efforts by home visitors to link mothers to effective mental health treatment, only 18% of depressed mothers received mental health services during that time. Third, depressed mothers required more support from home visitors (Stevens, Ammerman, Putnam, & Van Ginkel, 2002), and home visitors reported having more difficulty implementing the curricula given maternal symptomatology. Fourth, the overwhelming evidence for the negative effects of maternal depression on child development (Goodman & Gotlib, 2002) provided a sense of urgency to respond to this problem.

In the MDM, we developed and pilot tested In-Home Cognitive Behavior Therapy (IH-CBT), an intervention designed specifically for use in the context of home visitation. We chose to design a separately administered treatment because the evidence is clear that the best response to depression is treatment (which requires specialized training), and we also did not want to overburden home visitors with an additional task that deviates from their primary responsibility of providing home visitation. IH-CBT has four core features: (a) it is based on the empirically-supported CBT model for depression, (b) it is administered in the home to overcome barriers to obtaining effective treatment in clinic settings, (c) it is designed to address the specific needs and concerns of depressed first-time mothers, and (d) there are systematic procedures to ensure synergistic collaboration between the IH-CBT therapist and home visitor in order to maximize the benefits of both efforts.

A pre-post evaluation (Ammerman, Putnam, Stevens et al., 2005) of IH-CBT was carried out in 26 first-time mothers in home visitation who, during the first year of service, scored 20 or higher on the BDI-II and were diagnosed with major depression using a semi-structured interview. The sample had high pre-treatment BDI-II scores ($M = 30.35$), and exhibited histories of interpersonal trauma (73%), suicide attempts (35%), and hospitalizations (50%). IH-CBT was administered by a trained social worker over 17 weekly sessions, two of which were conducted with the home visitor present. Results indicated that 69% of mothers no longer met criteria for major depression at the end of treatment; an additional 15% were partially remitted. A 16-point reduction was found on the BDI-II ($F(1, 25)$ = 42.66, $p < .001$). Additional findings included decreased self-reported functional impairment, increased self-reported acceptance of and emotional closeness to the child, increased rate of home visiting during treatment period, and overall satisfaction with the program by mothers and home visitors. A detailed case study describing the clinical procedures of IH-CBT can be found in Ammerman et al. (2007).

CHALLENGES TO IMPLEMENTATION

While ECS has been effective in a number of areas, there have been significant challenges encountered. These challenges, we believe, are common in the prevention field, and warrant continued examination. Most large-scale, community-based home visitation programs operate in multiple sites. There are clear advantages to this structure: smaller agencies with strong ties to their local communities can be recruited, and geographic reach of services can be maximized. As the number of agencies increases, however, it becomes more difficult to maintain program fidelity, minimize interagency variability, and implement system-wide changes in an efficient and rapid manner. This phenomenon was also noted by Duggan et al. (2000), who found differences between sites in their evaluation of the Hawaii Healthy Start Program. Through eECS and our CQI efforts, ECS is focused on addressing these issues with some success, although a considerable amount of effort has been required to adequately meet this ongoing challenge.

An additional concern has been the management of outside forces and influences that undermine the primary mission of the program. There are numerous impediments to maintaining a focus on providing quality home visitation. Public and private funders have procedural and documentation requirements that are often time-consuming and require changes to data collection procedures and to information storage systems. ECS is especially vulnerable to this issue given that it operates in multiple regions and receives funding from several sources. The overall increase in the use of Web-based systems by government entities, funders, and other organizations requires that ECS find ways to adapt eECS to most efficiently interface with other Web-based systems. Management challenges increase proportionally with the size of the program, extent of geographic operations, and number of funders and oversight organizations.

Finally, it has become increasingly evident that there are a number of social and clinical issues that potentially undermine home visitation effectiveness. As previously noted, mothers who seek home visitation exhibit high rates of depression (Ammerman, Putnam, Altaye et al., 2007) and history of trauma (Stevens et al., 2002). Margie and Phillips (1999), in summarizing a national workshop on home visitation, reported that mental illness, domestic violence, and substance abuse are pervasive in populations enrolled in home visitation services. More recently, LeCroy and Whitaker (2005) found that 78.5% of home visitors reported working with mentally ill mothers in the last 30 days, 67.5% had encountered substance abuse and 64.6% had worked with mothers experiencing domestic violence during the same time period. Future research must identify ways of adapting or augmenting standard home visitation curricula to meet the needs of this sizable group of affected families.

REFERENCES

Ammerman, R. T., Bodley, A. L., Putnam, F. W., Lopez, W. L., Holleb, L. J., Stevens, J. et al. (2007). In-home cognitive behavior therapy for a depressed mother in a home visitation program. *Clinical Case Studies, 6*, 161-180.

Ammerman, R. T., Putnam, F. W., Altaye, M., Chen, L., Holleb, L. J., Stevens, J. et al. (2005). *Course of depression in first-time mothers in home visitation.* Unpublished manuscript, Cincinnati Children's Hospital Medical Center, Cincinnati, OH.

Ammerman, R. T., Putnam, F. W., Stevens, J., Holleb, L. J., Novak, A. L., & Van Ginkel, J. B. (2005). In-home cognitive behavior therapy for depression: An adapted treatment for first time mothers in home visitation. *Best Practices in Mental Health, 1*, 1-14.

Bavolek, S. J., & Keene, R. G. (1999). *Adult-Adolescent Parenting Inventory: AAPI-2.* Park City, UT: Family Development Resources, Inc.

Beck, A. T., Steer, R. A., & Brown, G. K. (1996). *Beck Depression Inventory-II Manual.* San Antonio: The Psychological Corporation.

Bickman, L., & Noser, K. (1999). Meeting the challenges in the delivery of child and adolescent mental health services in the next millennium: The continuous quality improvement approach. *Applied & Preventive Psychology, 8*, 247-255.

Caldwell, B. M., & Bradley, R. H. (1984). *Home observation for measurement of the environment administration manual* (Revised Edition). Little Rock, AK: Home Inventory.

Daro, D. A., & Harding, K. A. (1999). Healthy Families America: Using research to enhance practice. *The Future of Children, 9*, 152-176.

Deming, W. E. (1982). *Out of the crisis.* Cambridge, MA: Massachusetts Institute of Technology, Center for Advanced Engineering Study.

Domitrovich, C. E., & Greenberg, M. T. (2000). The study of implementation: Current findings from effective programs that prevent mental disorders in school-aged children. *Journal of Educational and Psychological Consultation, 11,* 193-221.

Donovan, E. F., Ammerman, R. T., Besh, J., Atherton, H., Khoury, J. C., Mekibib, A., Putnam, F. W., & Van Ginkel, J. B. (2007). Intensive home visiting is associated with decreased risk of infant death. *Pediatrics, 119,* 1145-1151.

Duggan, A., Windham, A., McFarlane, E., Fuddy, L., Rohde, C., Buchbinder, S. et al. (2000). Hawaii's Healthy Start Program of home visiting for at-risk families: Evaluation of family identification, family engagement, and service delivery. *Pediatrics, 105,* 250-259.

Frankenburg, W. K., Dodds, J., Archer, P., Bresnick, B., Maschka, P., Edelman, N. et al. (1996). *Denver II: Manuals* (2nd ed). Denver: Denver Developmental Materials.

Galano, J., Credle, W., Perry, D., Berg, S., Huntington, L., & Stief, E. (2001). Developing and sustaining a successful community prevention initiative: The Hampton Healthy Families Partnership. *Journal of Primary Prevention, 21,* 495-509.

Gomby, D. S. (1999). Understanding evaluations of home visitation programs. *The Future of Children, 9,* 27-43.

Goodman, S. H., & Gotlib, I. H. (Eds.) (2002). *Children of depressed parents: Mechanisms of risk and implications for treatment.* Washington, DC: American Psychological Association.

Guterman, N. B. (2001). *Stopping child maltreatment before it starts: Emerging horizons in early home visitation services.* Thousand Oaks, CA: Sage Publications.

Juran, J. M. (1992). *Juran on quality by design.* New York: The Free Press.

Karoly, L. A., Greenwood, P. W., Everingham, S. S., Hoube, J., Kilburn, M. R., Rydell, C. P. et al. (1998). *Investing in our children: What we know and don't know about the costs and benefits of early childhood intervention.* Santa Monica, CA: RAND.

Kopke, J. E., Carrozza, M., Witherow, B. A., Van Ginkel, J. B., Putnam, F. W., & Ammerman, R. T. (2003, November). *Every user succeeds.* Poster presented at the American Medical Informatics Association, Washington, DC.

Krug, S. (2000). *Don't make me think–A common sense approach to web usability.* Indianapolis: New Riders Publishing.

LeCroy, C. W., & Whitaker, K. (2005). Improving the quality of home visitation: An exploratory study of difficult situations. *Child Abuse & Neglect, 29,* 1003-1013.

Leventhal, J. M. (2005). Editorial: Getting prevention right: Maintaining the status quo is not an option. *Child Abuse & Neglect, 29,* 209-213.

Margie, N. G., & Phillips, D. A. (Eds.) (1999). *Revisiting home visiting: Summary of a workshop.* Washington, DC: National Academy Press.

Olds, D. L. (2003). Reducing program attrition in home visiting: What do we need to know? *Child Abuse & Neglect, 27,* 359-361.

Olds, D. L., Hill, P. L., O'Brien, R., Racine, D., & Moritz, P. (2004). Taking preventive intervention to scale: The Nurse-Family Partnership. *Cognitive & Behavioral Practice, 10,* 278-290.

Racine, D. P. (1998). *Replicating programs in social markets.* Philadelphia: Replication and Program Strategies, Inc.

Solberg, L. I., Brekke, M. L., Kottke, T. E., & Steel, R. P. (1998). Continuous quality improvement in primary care: What's happening? *Medical Care, 36*, 625-635.

Stevens, J., Ammerman, R. T., Putnam, F. G., & Van Ginkel, J. (2002). Depression and trauma history in first time mothers receiving home visitation. *Journal of Community Psychology, 30*, 551-564.

The Standish Group (1995). *The CHAOS report (1994)*. Retrieved June 16, 2005, www.standishgroup.com/sample_research/chaos_1994_4.php.

Thompson, L., Kropenske, V., Heinicke, C., Gomby, D., & Halfon, N. (2001). Home visiting: A service strategy to deliver Proposition 10 results. In H. Halfon, E. Shulman, & M. Hochstein (Eds.). *Building community systems for young children.* Los Angeles: UCLA Center for Healthier Children, Families and Communities.

doi:10.1300/J005v34n01_05

The Evaluation of Healthy Families Arizona:
A Multisite Home Visitation Program

Judy Krysik
Craig W. LeCroy

Arizona State University

SUMMARY. Healthy Families Arizona is a broadly implemented home visitation program aimed at preventing child abuse and neglect, improving child health and development, and promoting positive parent/child interaction. The program began as a pilot in two sites in 1991 and by 2004 had grown to 48 sites located in urban, rural, and tribal regions of the state. The unique administrative structure of the program and collaboration between evaluation and quality assurance have helped overcome many of the problems familiar to home visitation programs. This paper describes how a systematic focus to improve processes and outcomes has positioned the program for a randomized longitudinal study. Key components of the program are described and evaluation results are presented. doi:10.1300/J005v34n01_06 *[Article copies available for a fee from The Haworth Document Delivery Service: 1-800-HAWORTH. E-mail address: <docdelivery@haworthpress.com> Website: <http://www.HaworthPress.com> © 2007 by The Haworth Press, Inc. All rights reserved.]*

Address correspondence to: Judy Krysik, Mail Code 3920, 411 N. Central Avenue, Suite 800, Phoenix, AZ 85004 (E-mail: jkrysik@msn.com).

[Haworth co-indexing entry note]: "The Evaluation of Healthy Families Arizona: A Multisite Home Visitation Program." Krysik, Judy, and Craig W. LeCroy. Co-published simultaneously in *Journal of Prevention & Intervention in the Community* (The Haworth Press, Inc.) Vol. 34, No.1/2, 2007, pp. 109-127; and: *The Healthy Families America® Initiative: Integrating Research, Theory and Practice* (ed: Joseph Galano) The Haworth Press, 2007, pp. 109-127. Single or multiple copies of this article are available for a fee from The Haworth Document Delivery Service [1-800-HAWORTH, 9:00 a.m. - 5:00 p.m. (EST). E-mail address: docdelivery@haworthpress.com].

KEYWORDS. Healthy Families, home visitation, child abuse prevention, formative evaluation, quality improvement, summative evaluation

INTRODUCTION

Many of the programs developed to prevent child abuse and neglect in the past three decades involve home visitation. The rapid expansion of home visitation and its associated costs has focused attention on the effectiveness of this strategy. Evaluation plays two important roles with regard to home visitation. First is a formative role; evaluation is used to provide timely and relevant information to be used in quality improvement. Second is an important summative role; evaluation is used to determine overall effectiveness and accountability. The evaluation methods used for these two roles are different, and they have a preferred order that begins with pre- and quasi-experimental methods with the possibility of progressing to experimental methods.

Many of the stakeholders in home visitation including program administrators, advocates, and funders often refer to the summative role of evaluation. What they want from an evaluation is to be able to answer the question: Did the program work? Or, they want evidence to support what they already intuitively know, that, of course, the program works. There is plenty of evidence to suggest that in the absence of a process of quality improvement informed by evaluation, the formative evaluation role, that services will not be of sufficient quality, intensity, and fidelity to lead to the desired benefits for children and families (see, for example, Duggan et al., 2004). Moving too quickly to a summative evaluation of outcomes will likely result in disappointing, null results. There is also evidence, such as presented in this paper, to suggest that using evaluation to focus on quality improvement can lead to better services. This implies that programs will be much more likely to be able to demonstrate results when they are finally ready for summative evaluation. Randomized trials should not be attempted until it is demonstrated that the program is being implemented as planned, that there is sufficient attention to process, and that the program demonstrates–via quasi-experimental methods–the promise of effectiveness. Only then it is worthwhile to spend the time, effort, and money on an experimental study.

This article will discuss the ways in which evaluation can and should be used for both program improvement and accountability, drawing on the experience of the statewide evaluation of Healthy Families Arizona (HFAz) as an example. HFAz will be described, along with a history of the design and purpose of the formative evaluation process. Results will be summarized, beginning first with how the evaluation was used successfully for program management and quality improvement, and then to illustrate, via quasi-experimental approaches, that participating families appear to be benefiting. The paper concludes with a discussion of the plans for a randomized trial for the evaluation of HFAz, and some lessons distilled from this unique partnership between program administrators, quality assurance, and program staff.

HEALTHY FAMILIES ARIZONA

HFAz falls under the Healthy Families America (HFA) umbrella of home visitation programs and is one example of a broadly implemented statewide home visitation program. Unlike many home visitation programs, HFAz is not restricted to parents experiencing their first birth, but is open to all families. Participation in HFAz is voluntary and available for a lifetime maximum of five years. Consistent with the national model, the goals of HFAz are (a) to prevent child abuse and neglect, (b) to improve child health and development, and (c) to promote positive parent/child interaction.

HFAz is a relationship-based program. That means that the early development of a trusting, open, and constructive relationship between the parent and the home visitor is viewed as critical to the process. Eligible families are identified in select hospitals shortly after the birth of a child by a two-stage screening and assessment process conducted by a Family Assessment Worker. If the first screen is positive, the parent(s) can submit to a more detailed assessment interview based on the 10-item Family Stress Checklist (Abdin, 1995). If the score on the Family Stress Checklist is 25 or greater and space is available, the family is offered the program. Home visiting for new families is usually once a week for one hour, but can be more frequent if determined necessary. The home visitors are a mix of paraprofessionals and entry-level professionals. The number of home visits a family receives is based on a level system with well-defined criteria for increasing and decreasing intensity over the course of their involvement. The foci of the home visits vary and can address for example issues such as positive parent/child interaction, home safety, problem solving and coping skills; child development, health and nutrition; personal goals, emotional support, and referral services. Screening for child development occurs at regular intervals and children who are identified with a possible delay are referred for further assessment and services.

History of the HFAz Program

HFAz began in 1991 as a demonstration project in two counties and by 2000 had grown to 23 sites located in urban, suburban, rural and tribal regions of the state. A large legislative appropriation in mid-year 2004 more than doubled the program and for the first time the program began to enroll families in the prenatal period. Through its 48 sites, HFAz now reaches over 100 Arizona communities and is expected to serve 4,324 families in calendar year 2005. In addition to the home visitation services HFAz will provide to enrolled families in 2005, Family Assessment Workers will screen approximately 16,000 births and provide 2,700 family risk assessments. Information on local community resources will be offered to those families that are assessed ineligible for the program, as well as to those families that are offered the program but refuse.

A unique feature of HFAz is its strong, centralized administration. The Arizona Department of Economic Security (ADES) administers the program. In addition to contracting with local service providers to provide home visitation services, the ADES contracts out the evaluation and quality assurance components of the program. Training is housed within quality assurance and is a key component to the oversight and professional development of the program. A major benefit to the program has been 15 years of consistent leadership in central administration, quality assurance, and evaluation. The staff in these three components have worked as partners in the development and growth of HFAz.

Also guiding the program is a community-based, statewide steering committee with six standing committees focused on training, policies and procedures, credentialing, excellence, community partnerships, and advocacy. The statewide steering committee has representation from all levels of HFAz, including home visitors. Ad hoc committees are formed on an as-needed basis to examine special issues as they arise. For example, an ad hoc committee is currently addressing the issue of father involvement.

The state legislature also plays a major role in influencing the growth and development of the program. The legislature has control over the program's budget and despite 15 years of growth, HFAz has faced a yearly challenge to maintain its funding. In part, this is because funds for the program are appropriated on an annual basis. Only recently has HFAz been an actual line item in the state budget. The state legislature also has a history of legislating changes in the process and content of HFAz as described in the next section.

Legislated changes. Substantial changes have been made to the program in three areas as a result of changes in legislation. Early in the life of the program a concern was raised by some state legislators that HFAz was overly intrusive into families' personal lives. To deal with this concern the state passed legislation in the second year of the program that required families to consent to contact before HFAz staff could contact them. This meant that the hospital staff as opposed to the Family Assessment Worker had to ask parents permission to speak to them about the program. Protocols were also strengthened at this time to clearly communicate to families that the home visitors are required by law to report suspected incidents of child abuse and neglect to Child Protective Services (CPS). Undoubtedly these changes have reduced the number of families that would have otherwise been screened and offered the program.

The second legislated change involves the content of the program. The state legislature has recognized the value of HFAz as a vehicle to reach vulnerable families with young children. As a result, the legislators have, over time, added several expectations to HFAz's three child-centered goals. These include the expectation that the program will assist families to reduce illiteracy and dependency on welfare, encourage employment and self-sufficiency, require community service, and offer education on successful marriage. The achievement of these additional expectations is at least somewhat affected by the availability of local resources. Gains in maternal employment, for instance, are dependent upon the availability of job training and placement, educational opportunities, transportation, child care, and the local economy.

Each time the legislature adds new requirements, program content, oversight, training, and evaluation must also change. Flexibility in the evaluation is considered essential to ensure that the program is focusing on legislated changes and that corresponding outcome information will be available when it comes time to make funding decisions. Failure to monitor the legislated changes could lead to future budget cuts. In the past year the HFAz steering committee members have started a campaign to educate state legislators about HFAz. Another source of education for state legislators is the newly created newsletter, *Building Bridges: Linking Practice and Research on Home Visitation.* The quarterly newsletter that premiered in the spring of 2005 was developed to make information based on the best available research accessible to those who work in, and are responsible for, decision-making in home visitation programs. The newsletter is mailed to each state legislator as well as other stakeholders.

The third major change prompted by the legislature involves the program eligibility criteria. In 1999, assuming that the program was least effective for those with a history of CPS involvement, the legislature moved to deny families with prior CPS involvement participation in

HFAz. This change came about as a result of a finding by the State Office of the Auditor General. The 1998 Auditor General's report claimed that 27% of HFAz participants with prior CPS involvement were subject to a substantiated report of child abuse and neglect 6 months post program entry, compared to 5% of all HFAz participants, and 8% of a comparison group. The decision to change the eligibility criteria was made even though the report explicitly stated: "there are no comparable data that would allow for a conclusion of whether the program is effective or ineffective in reducing abuse among these [CPS involved] families" (1998, p. 4). It was not until 2004 that the state legislature reversed this decision, once again allowing families with prior CPS involvement to voluntarily participate in HFAz.

The Evaluation of HFAz

Since the inception of HFAz in 1991, LeCroy & Milligan Associates, Inc. have been contracted by ADES to conduct an annual evaluation which is summarized in a report to the state at the end of each calendar year. Beginning in 1995, and extending for a period of three years, the legislature also required the State Office of the Auditor General to conduct an independent evaluation of HFAz. This paper focuses on the methods and findings from the LeCroy & Milligan Associates, Inc. evaluations. For 15 years LeCroy & Milligan has collected data on every family that completes the HFAz two-stage screening and assessment process. The evaluation methods are described below in terms of those aimed at quality improvement and those used to assess program outcomes.

Methods for quality improvement. The administrators of HFAz have long been committed to a program improvement process driven by the information gained through ongoing formative evaluation. Throughout the history of HFAz, evaluation data have been used in conjunction with quality assurance and training to ensure that the program is achieving its goals and producing the expected outcomes. Early in the life of the evaluation it was recognized that the sites needed information beyond the aggregation of data that was presented in the annual evaluation reports. The initial response to this realization was to provide site-specific information in the appendices of the annual reports. In an effort to respond to the sites in a timelier manner and to make the data useable for quality assurance visits to the sites, LeCroy & Milligan Associates, Inc. moved to providing site-level data on a quarterly basis.

Since 1999 quarterly evaluation reports to each site have provided immediate feedback to ensure that processes that are not working well and outcomes that are less than expected receive immediate attention. Program specialists from the quality assurance team conduct a minimum of two visits to each site per year to provide follow-up on concerns highlighted in the quarterly evaluation reports. Problem areas identified through the quarterly reports are also followed-up by targeted training and technical assistance.

The evaluators work closely with the quality assurance and training staff to ensure that the site-level evaluation findings are useful to the sites and are used to influence practice. For instance, the reports include information on a range of process issues including the percentage of assessments completed, compliance with the required number of home visits and supervision standards, and worker retention and training. The reasons eligible families provide for declining the program are tracked and the sites receive quarterly data on acceptance rates that can be used in program improvement. The focus of the quarterly reports changes from time to time as new problem areas are identified and new practices are implemented. For instance, the most recent quarterly evaluation report tracks the enrollment of prenatal participants, a new practice implemented in 2004.

Pre-experimental methods are used periodically to take the pulse of the home visitor staff and the Family Assessment Workers. For instance, Internet surveys and focus groups have been used to obtain feedback from staff and supervisors on the measures, to collect data on the perceived impact of the program, and to discover the most challenging issues encountered by the home visitors. The evaluators take advantage of a two-day, statewide institute with mandated attendance for all HFAz staff to share evaluation findings and collect additional data as needed. In addition, a satisfaction survey of each enrolled family is conducted annually. On two occasions current and former participants were interviewed using a combination of in-person and telephone interviews to gather their perceptions on program services and perceived impact.

Methods to assess outcomes. The primary method used to determine outcomes is the assessment of change over time. Data collection points include entry to the program and 6-month intervals thereafter until termination or a period of 60 months. The second method is the use of a comparison group to evaluate between-group differences. In 1992, a comparison group of 302 at-risk families was recruited from hospitals located in areas demographically similar to those of HFAz program sites: those with relatively high rates of poverty and substantiated child abuse and neglect. Trained *family assessment workers* responsible for screening and recruitment collected similar demographic and risk data from mothers in the comparison group as they did for HFAz participants. The home visitors collected follow-up data from the comparison group mothers during visits to their homes at 6, 12 and 18 months.

Two statistically significant between-group differences were noted between the comparison group and HFAz participant group. First, scores on the Family Stress Checklist for mothers in the HFAz program from 1992 through 1996 were on average significantly higher, indicating greater risk among program participants compared to mothers in the comparison group. Second, scores on the Child Abuse Potential Inventory (CAPI; Milner, 1990), a screening scale for child physical abuse, revealed significantly greater potential for child physical abuse among HFAz participants in contrast to comparison group mothers. Although primary data collection activities with the comparison group ceased after 18 months, members of the comparison group were tracked in the CPS database to record substantiated incidents of child abuse and neglect until 1997.

RESULTS

This section presents select results from the 15 years of HFAz evaluation. It includes a description of the participants, quality improvement findings, and outcomes. The results are presented for select years because over time processes and outcome measures have changed making it difficult to compare across years.

Description of Participating Families

HFAz sites are strategically located in communities with high rates of child abuse and neglect, and poverty. Given the purposive nature of site selection and the two-stage screening process to determine eligibility it is no surprise that HFAz serves families with a number of risk factors. Table 1 presents data on select risk factors related to child abuse and neglect for the 800 families who enrolled in HFAz in the 9-month period beginning January 1, 2004.

The information in Table 1 shows that the typical HFAz participant who enrolled in the program was a low-income, single mother. Almost one-third of the participants were teenagers when their babies were born. Income level and pregnancy status qualifies the majority of program mothers for the state sponsored health insurance program; 90% of those with health-care insurance were enrolled in the state Medicaid program, the Arizona Health Care Cost Containment Program–AHCCCS. Still, a substantial percentage, 35%, received late, if any, prenatal care. Some

TABLE 1. Characteristics of Families Enrolling from January 1, 2004–September 30, 2004

Risk Factors	Percentage (N = 800)
Teen mother (less than 19 years)	31%
Married or cohabitating	18%
Less than high school education	
Mother	61%
Father	53%
Mother employed	15%
Late or no prenatal care	35%
Annual median income	$6,000
Health insurance	97%
Premature delivery (< 37 weeks)	13%
Low birth weight (< 2,500 grams)	12%
History of severe childhood abuse	
Mother	58%
Father	37%

Note. 575 fathers are represented in the data.

13% of HFAz mothers gave birth prematurely, and 12% of the babies were considered low birth weight. Around 58% of the 800 program mothers and 37% of the 575 fathers reported a history of severe childhood abuse.

Although the demographic information indicates several commonalities among HFAz participants, it also reveals a great deal of diversity. In this same cohort of 800 families, 56% of the mothers were Hispanic; 25% White, not Hispanic; 10% American Indian; 6% Black, and 3% of some other race or ethnicity. Diversity is also found in age; mothers ranged from 13 to 43 years-of-age and fathers from 14 to 67 years-of-age. For 51% of the mothers, the baby that made them eligible for the HFAz program was their first, whereas the other 49% of mothers had from one to seven children prior to their most recent birth.

The demographic data are used to tailor the HFAz program to the participants. For instance, because approximately one-third of the participants are teen mothers the instruments are evaluated for facility of use with adolescent girls. Information on the diversity of program participants is used to inform staff recruitment and training. Three specific challenges are the recruitment of Spanish speaking staff, translation of all program materials into Spanish, and increasing father involvement.

Results for Quality Improvement

The intense focus on quality and ensuring systematic processes has been recognized as an important aspect of improved program implementation. Prevent Child Abuse America (PCA America) and the Council on Accreditation implemented a statewide accreditation program for Healthy Families programs in 1999. The accreditation process credentials state systems as well as sites within state systems that document meeting nationally established research-based standards for quality service delivery and best practice standards for management and operations. HFAz was the first state system in the nation to receive that credential and was re-accredited in 2004 with no deferment or correction required.

One indicator of quality service is retention. If HFAz sites cannot maintain families in the program, then the families cannot benefit. Participant retention is a problem for many home visitation programs, with attrition rates often hovering around 50% in the first year (Daro et al., 2003; McCurdy et al., 1996; McGuigan et al., 2003). HFAz identified problems with retention in its first few years of operation and targeted it as an area of focus. As a result, retention rates have improved over time and are good relative to other voluntary home visitation programs. For instance, in 2001, only 4% of the 739 enrolled participants terminated involvement at three months, compared to 10% in Hawaii (Duggan et al., 2000). The average length of time families remain in HFAz also continues to increase. As shown in Table 2, the average number of days to termination has consistently increased from 2001 until 2004. In 2003 the average length of participation for those active in the program was over 2 years with 63% of the 2,356 active families having tenure of greater than 1 year.

Child and Family Outcomes

The next section presents data on the range of outcomes that are assessed in the program on an annual basis. As different measures have been used over the history of the evaluation, the data are presented for select periods of time. Also discussed is the manner in which the outcomes are operationalized and measured.

Child abuse and neglect. Child abuse and neglect is measured via an annual match of participant and comparison group names (both past and current) with the Arizona Child Protective Services Registry (CHILDS).

TABLE 2. Average Number of Days to Termination for Participants Terminating by Year

Year	Mean Days to Termination	N
2001	498	739
2002	596	669
2003	699	639
2004	805	629

Note. Average number of days to termination is calculated for those participants that the program considers engaged, that is, they must have completed four home visits.

Only substantiated incidents of child abuse and neglect are considered; reports classified as potential abuse and neglect are excluded. In addition, both HFAz program and comparison group children and their siblings if living in the same household are included in the match. Data on child abuse and neglect were made available annually from 1993 to 2005, with the exception of 1998 when the state department responsible for the data implemented a new automated information system.

One objective of HFAz is that 95% of participating families will not have a substantiated report of child abuse and neglect. The annual measurement of this objective from 1993 through 2004, excluding 1998 due to an absence of official data, has shown that this objective has consistently been met and exceeded. An analysis of CPS data for 1997 found 40 of 1,453 (2.8%) current and past HFAz families had at some time since 6-months post participation in HFAz been subject to at least one substantiated report of child abuse and neglect. In the same time period, 16 of the 302 comparison group families (5.2%) had received a substantiated report of child abuse and neglect. The difference between the two groups was statistically significant ($p < .05$), and notable given the surveillance bias in the HFAz group. Furthermore, a qualitative difference between the two groups in the types of substantiated incidents was also noted as seen in Table 3. The comparison group had a greater proportion of incidents classified by CPS as high-risk physical abuse than did the HFAz group, including one child death. The HFAz participant group, in contrast, had a greater proportion of incidents classified as neglect than the comparison group and no child deaths.

After 1998 when the Arizona legislature made the decision that HFAz would no longer serve any parent who had been subject to a substantiated report of child abuse or neglect, the overall rate of substantiated child abuse and neglect incidents in the HFAz group dropped substantially.

TABLE 3. Comparison of Substantiated Abuse and Neglect Incidents as of March 1997

Type of Incident	HFAz (N = 40)	Comparison (N = 16)
High risk physical abuse	12%	34%
Low risk physical abuse	6%	7%
High risk neglect	23%	13%
Medium risk neglect	24%	26%
Low risk neglect	35%	20%

This is because a high-risk group, those with a history of CPS involvement, was eliminated from the program. For instance, substantiated child abuse and neglect rates for HFAz participants were 0.8% in 2001 and 0.7% in 2002 and 2003. It is expected that as a result of the 2004 policy change to again serve parents regardless of past CPS involvement that there will be a corresponding increase in the percentage of families with substantiated child abuse and neglect reports.

Parental stress. A between-group comparison was also conducted using the Parental Stress Index (PSI; Abdin, 1995). The PSI is a reliable and validated measure used extensively in research and evaluation. The PSI asks parents to rate the stress they are experiencing in 11 areas including sense of competence, parental attachment, feeling restricted in role, depression, relationship with spouse, social isolation, health, parental distress, difficult child, social support, and parental self-efficacy. The PSI was administered at entry and again at 6 and 18 months.

Over multiple years, HFAz parents have consistently shown significant improvements on the PSI from entry into the program to 6, 12, and 18 months. Significant improvements have been noted in mothers' sense of competence, parental attachment, social support, parental efficacy, and perceived health. Significant decreases have been noted in depression, feeling restricted in their parental role, parental distress, social isolation and difficult parent/child interactions. Examining within-group changes is limited, however, because factors other than the program could be influencing the change, for example, the age of the child. To address this problem the PSI was also administered to the comparison group of 302 new mothers to examine between-group changes. Whereas the HFAz group showed significant improvements on 10 of the 11 parental stress subscales, the comparison group did not. In fact, in the period from 3 weeks after birth to 6 months, data from the independent comparison group showed a significant negative progression on the same 10 of 11 subscales on which the HFAz group showed significant improvements. The one area not showing a significant difference for either HFAz or comparison group was relationship with spouse.

The PSI was replaced in 2005 with the Healthy Families Parenting Inventory (HFPI), a new instrument developed by LeCroy & Milligan Associates, Inc., with significant input from HFAz supervisors and home visitors. The PSI was replaced because the home visitors had long-standing concerns that several of the items did not fit with the strength-based approach of HFAz. Home visitors generally disliked administering the PSI and therefore only completed it to comply with data requirements. After piloting and testing an initial item-pool for reliability and factorial validity, the HFPI was revised and implemented. The resulting instrument has a total of 67 items each measured on a 5-point scale and is divided into 10 subscales. The HFPI subscales include social support, depression, mobilizing resources, parent/child behavior, parenting competence, problemsolving, personal care, commitment to parent role, home environment, and parenting efficacy.

Informal feedback from the home visitors suggests that the HFPI is consistent with the HFAz practice model. Instead of feeling like the instrument is distracting from what they are trying to achieve with participating families, the home visitors report that the HFPI helps to focus their work, guides conversations with families, and assists with goal-setting. An assessment of the validity of the HFPI using confirmatory factor analysis is currently underway.

Developmental screening. Early identification of developmental delays is attempted through the administration of the Ages and Stages Questionnaire (Squires, Bricker, & Potter, 1997), a developmental screening instrument. Home visitors use the ASQ to conduct developmental screens at 6-month intervals all the way to 60 months. If the ASQ results suggest a developmental delay, the intent is for the HFAz home visitor to assist in linking the family to early intervention services. Of the children screened for a developmental delay in 2004, 5% screened positive at 6 months of age ($N = 440$), 11% at 12 months ($N = 280$), 18% at 18 months ($N = 203$), 22% at 24 months ($N = 200$), and 15% at 30 months ($N = 185$).

Initially the completion rate of developmental screening was low; about 75% for the first screen, dropping to around 12% at 12 months. The rate of completion improved dramatically once quality assurance data were provided to the sites. Efforts were also made to provide the home visitors with additional ASQ training. Data for 2004 show a 93% ASQ completion rate. Quarterly evaluation reports to the sites, training, and follow-up by the quality assurance team were essential in improving compliance with ASQ administration. In the past year the evaluators have started to monitor referrals to early intervention services for developmental delays, including who made the referral, whether or not services were received as a result of the referral, and the reason if services were not provided. There are no comparison data currently available on developmental screening.

Safety practices. Since 1998 safety practices have been measured at 2, 6, and 12 months, with a 25-item Child Safety Checklist developed specifically for the program. The checklist includes such items as covered electrical outlets; smoke alarms; car seats; storage of scissors, knives, lighters, matches, and poisons; water safety practices; availability of emergency phone numbers; outdoor supervision; and food storage. A second checklist has recently been developed for use in the prenatal component of HFAz.

In 2004 improvements in home safety from 2 to 12 months included increases in several safety practices. For instance, covering electrical outlets increased from 46% to 76%; the use of gates increased from 9% to 16%; locking away poisons increased from 83% to 94%, and stove protection increased from 90% to 98%. These findings indicate that at the 12-month assessment point, many HFAz families are practicing the child safety procedures recommended by the program. It is expected, however, that these common home safety practices would increase as children become more mobile with age. This is why a comparison or control group is needed to put the safety data into context.

Health practices. Medical outcomes are based on parent self-report. Parents are routinely asked questions on immunizations and linkage to a medical doctor. All medical information is updated every 6 months. The percentage of HFAz families reporting a primary care physician who provides health care to the infant has been consistently high at all observation points. Data from all years show that upward of 97% of infants were linked to a primary care physician at 2, 6, and 12 months. This finding may result because approximately 97% of HFAz mothers have some form of health insurance upon entry to the program.

The ability to affect outcomes through collaboration between evaluation and quality assurance is perhaps best demonstrated in the findings on immunization. In 1994, the immunization rate for HFAz program 2-year-olds was only slightly higher than the comparable state immunization rate, 50% compared to 46% respectively; and much lower than desired. It was determined that the low rate of immunization among program children was likely a factor of both poor documentation and poor compliance. In 1995, HFAz targeted immunization as a focus for improvement.

Once individual sites started to receive quarterly evaluation data on completed immunizations, data collection and reporting improved, as did attention to immunization in the home visits. In July 2000, quarterly evaluation reports to the sites were changed from presenting aggregate immunization completion rates to listing all immunizations completed by family identification number. By 2004, the HFAz immunization completion rate was 91% (N = 913), 14 percentage points higher than the state rate of 77%. The Arizona Department of Health Services calculates completion to include four diphtheria, tetanus and pertussis, three polio, and one measles-containing vaccination by age 2.

Drug and alcohol screening. Screening and referral for families experiencing drug and alcohol problems was implemented in 1998. The home visitor administered the CAGE, a standardized alcohol-screening instrument plus some additional questions to detect drug problems. A positive drug or alcohol screen results in a referral for treatment. The percentage of families who screened positive for alcohol or drugs in 2002 was 7% at 2 months (N = 518), 4% at 6 months (N = 434), 6% at 12 months (N = 386), and 5% at 18 months (N = 268). A very similar pattern of low positive rates was repeated in 2003 and 2004. Additional data, however, show that in 1994 the home visitors provided information or educational materials about substance abuse to 98 of 119 families at 12 months, and made referrals to a substance abuse service provider or self-help resource such as Alcoholics Anonymous for 11% or 14 families. This suggested that the CAGE was not identifying alcohol problems to the extent that they may exist. Recent research has shown that the CAGE is less sensitive and reliable with women and teens than with men (O'Hare & Tran, 1997). The HFAz home visitors reported a perception that the CAGE encouraged socially desirable answers and were concerned that some items were static as opposed to dynamic indicators. Questions that ask *did you ever*, for instance, cannot capture change. As a result, the CAGE was replaced in 2005 with the CRAFFT, a screening instrument that has shown good reliability with teens (Knight et al., 2002). Informal data from the home visitors support a preference for using the CRAFFT over the CAGE.

Maternal life course outcomes. Although HFAz focuses on parent-child interaction as a primary goal, evaluation of the program since 1998 has also included maternal life course outcomes. This change was driven by new legislation that coincided with welfare reform and added expectations for HFAz in the area of self-sufficiency.

Parent self-report measures of life course outcomes include the amount of time between pregnancies and gains in education and employment. In 2002, mothers' employment including full- and part-time at 12 months was 41% ($N = 547$), up from 16% at entry. In 2002, 11% of 533 HFAz participating mothers were enrolled full-time in school at 12 months, and an additional 7.3% were enrolled part-time. Also in 2002, 12% or 254 participants ($N = 2,099$) reported a subsequent pregnancy; 43% of those became pregnant within 1 to 2 years of program involvement. In 2004, 15% or 320 program participants ($N = 2,137$) became pregnant while enrolled in the program; of these, 30% were 18 years of age or younger and 32% were pregnant within the first year. The evaluators have recommended that the program focus on the issue of delaying subsequent births, with a special emphasis on teens. There are not comparison data to place these findings in context.

The Next Challenge

Program effectiveness is a concern shared by all parties interested in the prevention of child abuse and neglect. For 15 years the results of the independent evaluation using a combination of pre- and quasi-experimental methods have been mostly favorable toward HFAz. As a result of the unique partnership between evaluation, quality assurance, and central administration, HFAz has grown and improved. The program has also benefited from the lessons learned in other evaluations of home visitation programs and from participation in the national network of HFA. For instance, as a result of evaluation findings by Duggan et al. (2004), HFAz is working toward a clearer focus on outcomes that encompass the most salient risk factors for child abuse and neglect. This is being accomplished through the development of a program logic model that links specific outcomes with the resources necessary for achievement and the measures necessary to document change.

The question remains unanswered, however, as to whether or not an equivalent group of families would obtain the same or better results without the assistance of HFAz. Ideally it would be helpful to answer this question by generalizing from existing controlled studies. Experimental design in the context of a broadly implemented community-based program such as HFAz is costly and difficult to manage. Implementing randomization is difficult because of ethical objections related to denying needy families potentially helpful services. Unfortunately, the ability to generalize from existing experimental studies of home visitation is complicated. Existing literature reviews and meta-analyses of home visiting programs have come to conflicting conclusions. This is not surprising, given that any one review has to contend with the apples and oranges that form the literature on home visitation. Home visiting is a means of service delivery, not a program model. Literature reviews and meta-analyses often combine results from studies of home visiting programs that differ in their goals, program models, curricula, populations served, communities involved, service mix, duration, and intensity. In addition to differences in structure and content of the programs reviewed, there are differences in pilot versus scaled-up research, the research methods themselves, and the administrative auspices of the services.

Concerns over the effectiveness of HFAz have been raised mostly in response to published studies that have shown mixed evidence of program effectiveness. Since HFAz has become such a big budget item it has attracted and will continue to attract substantially more attention than in the past. This has led program administrators to the conclusion that they need to embark on a controlled, longitudinal evaluation. The controlled evaluation was planned and participant recruitment began November 2005. The study will go beyond the current annual evaluation of the program in the measurement of several domains including child maltreatment.

Evidence on child abuse and neglect is only as good as the method by which the variable is identified (Cicchetti, 2004). Relying on CPS reports as an indicator of child abuse and neglect is problematic in several respects. First, CPS-substantiated child abuse and neglect incidents are low occurring events; second, many incidents of child abuse and neglect go unreported. Duggan and colleagues (2004) found that while substantiated CPS reports were low, self-reported abusive and neglectful behaviors were common. A more expansive definition of child abuse and neglect is consistent with the preventive intent of HFAz and its focus on healthy growth and development. A broader conceptualization will move the focus away from whether or not the family came to the attention to CPS to focus on the interaction between the parent and child. The controlled evaluation will also examine the degree that the home visitors are addressing the most salient risk factors related to child abuse and neglect.

DISCUSSION

HFAz is one of many programs in the country that implements the Healthy Families model of home visitation endorsed and supported by PCA America. Collaboration between the evaluation and the quality assurance teams has been instrumental in improving HFAz processes and outcomes. The evaluation has evolved over the life of the program to be flexible to changes legislated by the state and to concerns of the home visitors that measurement should guide and not drive the program.

Data collected through quasi-experimental means have suggested a favorable program impact. For instance, the between-group differences on substantiated rates of child abuse and neglect suggest a positive program impact, especially in light of the significantly lower risk for child abuse and neglect at baseline favoring the comparison group over the HFAz participant group. These data are supported by positive changes in parental stress in the first year after birth among program participants, and the negative progression of parental stress in the comparison group. The evaluation findings also suggest that home visitation can accomplish a broad range of goals beyond a decrease in child abuse and neglect. Some of these benefits include increased rates of immunization compared to the state, and the early detection of developmental delays in childhood. Other outcomes such as linkage to a medical home, mental health and substance abuse services; improved home safety practices; and maternal life course outcomes such as education, employment, and delaying subsequent birth need to be assessed in relation to a control group. Improvement in these areas cannot be meaningfully interpreted without reference to a control group.

The formative evaluation of HFAz has provided a window of opportunity to address the challenges that explain the variations in outcomes across controlled studies of home visitation. These include, for example, poorly developed program theory, poor participant retention, a lack of fidelity to the program model, insufficient training, and the use of measures that are not consistent with program objectives. Subjecting programs to randomized trials without adequate attention to process and outcome problems can provide a disservice to the program and is damaging to the reputation of the program model on a broader scale.

Experience from HFAz suggests that program administrators and evaluators need to be proactive at working with the state legislators. For instance, HFAz has launched an education campaign to inform freshman legislators about the program and carry out advocacy work prior to and during budget negotiations. The evaluators have taken the lead in providing the home visitation and stakeholder communities, including legislators, with up-to-date research on home visitation through a quarterly newsletter.

An important aspect of the evaluation of HFAz is that the data that are gathered are analyzed and directed toward multiple purposes. Some of the data are used to provide timely information to the sites through quarterly evaluation reports. The quality assurance team uses these data in targeted training efforts and technical assistance. Other data are aggregated and provide an overall picture of program outcome for the state. The planned longitudinal, controlled study will not only provide information on program effectiveness, but will allow the piloting of a number of new measures in domains that are not currently addressed in the ongoing evaluation. This experience should inform and lead to improvements in measurement for the ongoing evaluation, and ultimately improved services and outcomes for participating families.

REFERENCES

Abdin, R. L. (1995). *The parenting stress index*. Odessa, FL: Psychological Assessment Resources.

Cicchetti, D. (2004). An odyssey of discovery: Lessons learned through three decades of research on child maltreatment. *American Psychologist, 59*, 731-740.

Daro, D., McCurdy, K., Falconnier, L., & Stonjanovic, D. (2003). Sustaining new parents in home visitation services: Key participant and program factors. *Child Abuse and Neglect, 27*, 1101-1125.

Duggan, A., McFarlane, E., Fuddy, L., Burrell, L., Higman, S. M., Windham, A. et al. (2004). Randomized trial of a statewide home visiting program: Impact in preventing child abuse and neglect. *Child Abuse and Neglect, 28*, 597-622.

Duggan, A., Windham, A., McFarlane, E., Fuddy, L., Rohde, C., Buchbinder, S. et al. (2000). Hawaii's Healthy Start Program of home visiting for at-risk families: Evaluation of family identification, family engagement and service delivery. *Pediatrics, 105*, 250-259.

Knight, J. R., Sherritt, L., Shrier, L. A., Harris, S. K., & Chang, G. (2002). Validity of the CRAFFT substance abuse screening test among adolescent clinic patients. *Archives of Pediatric & Adolescent Medicine, 156*, 607-614.

McCurdy, K., Hurvis, S., & Clark, J. (1996). Engaging and retaining families in child abuse prevention programs. *The APSAC Advisor, 9*, 3-8.

McGuigan, W. M., Katzev, A. R., & Pratt, C. C. (2003). Multi-level determinants of retention in a home-visiting child abuse prevention program. *Child Abuse and Neglect, 27*, 363-380.

Milner, J. (1990). *An interpretive manual for the Child Abuse Potential Inventory*. DeKalb, IL: Psytec.

O'Hare, T., & Tran, T. V. (1997). Predicting problem drinking in college students: Gender differences and the CAGE questionnaire. *Addictive Behavior, 22*(1), 13-21.

Squires, J., Bricker, D., & Potter, L. (1997). Revision of a parent-completed development screening tool: Ages and Stages Questionnaire. *Journal of Pediatric Psychology, 22*, 313-328.

State of Arizona, Office of the Auditor General (1998). Annual evaluation: Healthy Families Pilot program report #98-1. Retrieved April 10, 2005, from http://www. auditorgen.state.az.us/Reports/state_Agencies/Agencies/Economic%20Security, %20Department%20of/Performance/98-1/98-1.pdf

doi:10.1300/J005v34n01_06

The Promise of Primary Prevention
Home Visiting Programs:
A Review of Potential Outcomes

Beth S. Russell

Worcester State College

Preston A. Britner

University of Connecticut

Jennifer L. Woolard

Georgetown University

SUMMARY. Home visitation (HV) is a promising service delivery model, despite a history of mixed documented results. Compiling results on the promising family and child development outcomes in the HV literature has utility for current programs and those under development. We review traditional outcomes (e.g., child maltreatment prevention) from the literature on HV, but we also present nontraditional outcomes (e.g., community connection) that may be relevant for future evaluations. Programs that document their implementation and study their outcomes through a

Address correspondence to: Beth S. Russell, PhD, Department of Psychology, Worcester State College, 486 Chandler Street, Worcester, MA 01602 (E-mail: bethsrussell@gmail.com).

[Haworth co-indexing entry note]: "The Promise of Primary Prevention Home Visiting Programs: A Review of Potential Outcomes." Russell, Beth S., Preston A. Britner, and Jennifer L. Woolard. Co-published simultaneously in *Journal of Prevention & Intervention in the Community* (The Haworth Press, Inc.) Vol. 34, No.1/2, 2007, pp. 129-147; and: *The Healthy Families America® Initiative: Integrating Research, Theory and Practice* (ed: Joseph Galano) The Haworth Press, 2007, pp. 129-147. Single or multiple copies of this article are available for a fee from The Haworth Document Delivery Service [1-800-HAWORTH, 9:00 a.m. - 5:00 p.m. (EST). E-mail address: docdelivery@haworthpress.com].

Available online at http://jpic.haworthpress.com
doi:10.1300/J005v34n01_07

thoughtful, planned process may capture important and much needed infor-
mation on strengthening families through HV. doi:10.1300/J005v34n01_07
[Article copies available for a fee from The Haworth Document Delivery Ser-
vice: 1-800-HAWORTH. E-mail address: <docdelivery@haworthpress.com>
Website: <http://www.HaworthPress.com> © 2007 by The Haworth Press, Inc.
All rights reserved.]

KEYWORDS. Home visitation, child abuse, intervention, program
evaluation

INTRODUCTION

Home visiting (HV) programs provide services in the form of social
support, parent education, and crisis intervention for the promotion of
healthy pregnancies, infants and families, and the prevention of negative
outcomes such as child abuse and neglect. Because services are brought to
and offered in the home, home visitors may be able to reach families not able
to access family support programs (Garbarino & Kostelny, 1994; Sweet &
Appelbaum, 2004). HV programs are guided by several assumptions that
are shared with other family support programs: (a) parents are usually the
most consistent caregivers for their children; (b) parents can respond positively and effectively to their children when parents are given the knowledge,
skills, and support necessary; and, (c) parents' emotional and physical needs
must be met in order for them to be effective parents (Reppucci, Britner, &
Woolard, 1997).

HV programs represent a promising preventive service option for meeting the U.S. Advisory Board on Child Abuse and Neglect's (ABCAN) goal
of "strengthening urban, suburban, and rural neighborhoods as environments for children and families" (Melton & Barry, 1994, p. 8). It was in large
part this goal of protecting the health and safety of the nation's children
through a neighborhood-based protection system (Thompson & Ontai,
2000) that prompted the proliferation of HV programs in the last decade.
Today, it is still a major focus of these programs to increase the health and
safety of participating families.

In this paper, we will focus on child and family development issues
related to more broad-based, preventive HV models in the U.S. We then
review research findings on traditional (e.g., child maltreatment prevention) and nontraditional (e.g., community connection) outcome variables
associated with HV models. We conclude with recommendations for

future practice and research. This review should give the interested reader: (a) a sense of the strength of HV as a prevention strategy; (b) a glimpse of the current (limited) research base of how HV may influence a variety of child and family outcomes; and (c) a clearer understanding that not all HV programs are alike, even within the HFA network, and thus the need to understand "process" before attempting to assess "outcomes."

KEY IMPLEMENTATION/PROCESS VARIABLES

Impediments to evaluating the "effectiveness" of HV include the wide variety of program models, target groups, parents' demographic character-istics, social network ties, home visitors' training, parent-home visitor rela-tionship parameters, program length and setting, recruitment and retention strategies, research methods employed to date, and the variety of outcome variables studied (Geeraert, Van den Noortgate, Grietens, & Onghena, 2004; Sweet & Appelbaum, 2004). This flexibility in implementation may be viewed as a strength of many HV programs, in that it permits the tailoring of services to the unique contextual community or family needs. However, with so many variables, it is difficult to isolate what constitutes a program model, much less evaluate its effectiveness.

With some notable exceptions (e.g., Olds et al., 1999; Daro & Harding, 1999; Duggan, McFarlane et al., 2004), research has been methodologi-cally flawed. Most evaluation studies consist of simple pre- and post-test designs without a control group, and represent important *initial* steps in establishing the efficacy of the programs. It is unclear to what extent pro-grams are implemented according to the curricula, getting through to par-ents, resulting in desired changes in parental and child behavior, and having a lasting impact. The database is limited, and the variety of pro-grams makes generalizability difficult; overall, answers are lacking to questions of program effectiveness (Sweet & Appelbaum, 2004). These broad conclusions are often built upon meta-analytic reviews of previous work, which by necessity are constrained to narrow inclusion criteria. Although the meta-analytic approach is valuable, this paper uses a much broader lens to explore overall effectiveness HV as a service delivery method.

Program Fidelity

The degree to which programs or curricula are modified (versus strictly adhered to) is an important area of study in evaluating effects, given the wide variety of implementation practices in the field. As Chaffin (2004) notes, meta-analyses of HV programs are limited by the fact that so few programs have maintained the same structure or research design over time. Programs often change as they expand from demonstration projects to larger-scale implementation across sites, which may vary as communities and in the way they implement the intervention (e.g., Leventhal, 2001). Research must identify core components of programs that are required for prevention program fidelity, while allowing other components to vary.

Risk Level

Most HV programs are restricted to risk groups (Sweet & Appelbaum, 2004). Referrals to some existing HV programs result from being labeled at risk by virtue of age, marital status, socioeconomic status, or previous referral to a child protection agency. Although many of these characteristics are associated with child maltreatment, the risk of false positives is quite high (Leventhal, Garber, & Brady, 1989). Incorrectly labeling a family as being in need of services may lead to unintended negative consequences.

Thus, a universal approach to home-visiting, in which services are offered to all families in communities, would circumvent this problem and forever remove the "stigma of eligibility" present in many social service programs (Reppucci et al., 1997). A true "systems of care" primary (or universal) prevention approach would include services for all families and be assured of reaching those most in need of services. Healthy Families America® (HFA; Daro & Harding, 1999), for example, is an "entirely voluntary" program that is aimed at supporting and aiding *all* parents with their own child-rearing goals. However, there are HFA programs that extend services to all families "at risk for child abuse and neglect" (Galano et al., 2001), focusing intervention efforts to a specific subset of a given community's families.

Client risk is an essential "process" variable. Depending on the outcome of interest and the nature of the HV program, riskier groups may be less likely to participate, although they are in greater need of the services (Garbarino & Kostelny, 1994; McCurdy & Daro, 2001). Even within a program, client risk may differentially influence services and outcomes.

Intensity of Services

Olds et al. (1999) report that HV programs with clear structure, frequent person-to-person contact, and fewer invasive procedures seem to be the most successful. In fact, most reviews of HV and parenting literatures call for intensive, sustained contact with clients. However, a recent review of 1,601 participants in family preservation and family support programs found few differences in child maltreatment outcomes across intensity of services, as well as client risk levels, program types, and program completion status (Chaffin, Bonner, & Hill, 2001). Neither Parents as Teachers (PAT) nor HFA participants fared well, and neither program addressed needs of high-risk clients. The study's authors note that it was hard to evaluate process variables, like fidelity of implementation, in interpreting the outcomes. In a meta-analysis of family wellness programs, MacLeod and Nelson (2000) found very low effect sizes on child maltreatment prevention for HV programs with 12 or fewer visits and less than a 6-month duration. When Healthy Families/Healthy Start programs have controlled for the dose of service delivered to program participants, results have been mixed (Duggan, McFarlane et al., 2004).

Community Focus

The need for community change is perhaps most clearly illustrated with extreme examples such as crime-ridden violent neighborhoods that present safety risks to children. However, the need to focus on community does not arise from extreme examples alone. A community development approach builds supports for families into the community structure so that families can marshal additional resources (e.g., social capital) to overcome risk and foster a healthy developmental environment (Furstenberg & Hughes, 1997). Ideally over time, family support (both formal and informal) becomes typical of the way communities operate.

Structural and compositional characteristics of communities may concentrate risks for some families in particular locations and set the macro-level context in which families function. The degree of social organization in a community has an important effect on that community's ability to achieve shared goals such as healthy family development (Sampson & Morenoff, 1997). A community with weak or suboptimal structural and compositional characteristics will likely have a weaker social organization, which in turn creates a context that is less supportive of child and family well-being. An organized, well-functioning community can be characterized in terms of the organizational participation and empowerment of its citizens, the informal social networks that link citizens to each other, and the collective supervision of youth by all community members. A community with clarity and consensus about norms and values can promote and support healthy growth among children and families. Norms of valuing children, supporting families, and communal responsibility for well-being, when present, can create a context that enables families to reach their potential (Furstenberg & Hughes, 1997; see Daro et al., this volume).

Process Variables Associated with Success

Voluntary programs such as Healthy Families/Healthy Start appear promising as strategies to prevent child abuse and neglect and may be a viable alternative to a coercive child protection system centered on investigation and treatment. As Wolfe et al. (1995) point out, early interventions that employ more personal service provision methods (like HV) are the most successful programs at reaching the highest-risk participants.

Reppucci, Britner, and Woolard (1997) found that family support and prevention programs that served families most successfully had several characteristics in common, including long-term and intensive services and program staff competence in leadership, relationship building within the program and among community service agencies, fund-raising, long-term planning, and program flexibility given a range of family needs. According to Wandersman and Florin (2003), prevention science has identified nine characteristics of prevention programs (programs not identified as parent education specifically) consistently associated with efficacy; these include "comprehensive, varied teaching methods, sufficient dosage, research based/theory driven, positive relationships, appropriately timed, socioculturally relevant, outcome evaluation, and well-trained staff" (p. 445). Of the nine qualities identified, those relevant to program implementation have received the most attention in the broader parent education literature.

Published evaluations of multiple models of parent education have demonstrated the need for well-trained service providers (Nation et al., 2003; Olds et al., 1998; Wandersman & Florin, 2003). Meta-analyses of prevention programming available to families with young children find that parent education that is most successful in creating change in parent or child outcomes employs *professional* educators (i.e., those with professional degrees and formal training; Layzer et al., 2001; Sweet & Appelbaum, 2004). In a 15-year follow-up, Olds et al. (1998) found that those families who worked with Registered Nurse Practitioner home visitors benefited more than did those families who worked with paraprofessional home visitors across a variety of outcomes.

TRADITIONAL OUTCOMES ASSOCIATED
WITH HOME VISITING PROGRAMS

Efficacy studies for HV programs have included traditional family and early childhood outcomes and, in some cases, several nontraditional measures. We begin with a review of four types of traditional, individual outcomes: formal supports/services; child maltreatment prevention; school readiness; and, the prevention of antisocial or delinquent behavior. It is noteworthy that many child and family outcomes are interconnected. We have drawn lines between outcomes for ease of organization, not to suggest clear boundaries between domains.

Formal Supports/Services

Perhaps the most fundamental component of most HV programs is the connection of families to services of which they might not have been aware. Beyond services, the nature of HV adds an element of support to the family through providing a trained professional to listen, observe, teach, and be available to a family that might previously have been isolated. The formal services most often include medical care, parenting programs, and mental health provisions. This section will focus on the discussion of health outcomes associated with family participation in HV models of prevention.

Improved Health Outcomes

HV programs continue to place a major focus on improving the health of participating families. As such, nearly all programs have, at a minimum, processes in places to refer parents and children to health-care services on a preventive and emergent basis. Most programs include inter-agency ties to local departments of child welfare and hospitals, but many also include referral processes to ensure that expectant mothers receive some degree of prenatal care, and that infants and young children receive preventive care.

It is important to note that in all cases families at greater risk benefited most. HV has reduced negative birth outcomes through increasing prenatal care service utilization and decreasing the number of poor maternal health habits during pregnancy. These negative birth outcomes include fewer low birth weight babies, pre-term births, drug dependent babies, and fewer malnourished newborns (Daro & Harding, 1999; Eckenrode, 2000; Olds et al., 1999). Each of these risk factors can contribute to developmental delays including impaired cognition, language acquisition, and social-emotional development (Emig, 2000).

HV stands to improve the health of families and young children when home visitors are trained to intervene in relevant areas and when participating families are in need of health-specific intervention. Whereas some studies have found that paraprofessional home visitors may struggle to make adequate linkages between families in need and available community resources (Duggan, Fuddy et al., 2004), home visitors with sufficient training can make referrals, remind parents of appointments, and support families in seeking out quality care for their children. Ultimately home visitors cannot ensure that these children will experience lasting, improved health; parents must be dedicated to ensuring and protecting their children's health. However, HV initiatives can move beyond a client-based service delivery model to develop a community context that supports parents, increasing the likelihood that parents can in turn meet their children's health need (see Daro et al., this volume).

Child Maltreatment Prevention

Recent, broader definitions of child protection programs include voluntary, neighborhood-based, child-centered, and family-focused programs, as proposed by U.S. ABCAN (Melton & Barry, 1994). HV programs that promote child and family welfare fit this description. These programs provide voluntary educational and support services, and most often operate apart from the formal child protection system.

Services offered through HV programs depend on the skill level of the visitor and the program's underlying assumptions about preventing negative outcomes and promoting the well-being of families. For example, if a program assumes that isolation and psychosocial stress are causes of child maltreatment, the visitor may fulfill a primarily supportive, social role (Olds & Kitzman, 1990). In contrast, if the assumption is that parents lack adequate knowledge of child development, the visitor may serve as an educator and model appropriate interaction with the infant. As the visitor's role complexity increases, the education and training level of the visitor must also increase (Reppucci et al., 1997).

Most HV programs have failed to show reductions in maltreatment rates or even assess child abuse and neglect as an outcome (Chaffin et al., 2001; Duggan, McFarlane et al., 2004). Some relevant data are available, however (see Harding et al., this volume; Krysik & LeCroy, this volume; Martin et al., this volume). In their meta-analysis of 40 secondary prevention programs for parents of young children, Geeraert et al. (2004) found a significant decrease in child and family risks and in rates of child abuse; there were no differences in effect sizes (which ranged from .20 to .38) between HFA and other prevention programs. (For additional results on HV impact on child maltreatment, see Wolfe et al., 1995; Olds et al.,1999; Eckenrode et al., 2000; and Olds & Kitzman, 1990.)

HV programs need to be designed with a focus on the ecology of the family during pregnancy and early childhood. In other words, HV must occur frequently and extend over a period of time long enough to be able to address the factors that influence child and parental outcomes. Several studies support timing and duration of home visits as a crucial factor, with early and extended contact between mother and visitor contributing to successful intervention. Only after daily crises (e.g., threat of eviction) in the lives of poor families were resolved could the mothers' attention become focused on parenting and health issues. In turn, home visitors often became valued resources and advocates.

School Readiness

The majority of HV research has focused on children from birth through the first 2 or 3 years of life. As such, data on children as they enter school at age five are sparse. There is evidence to support the supposition that other potential outcomes associated with HV (i.e., utilization of both community and personal resources, reduction of child maltreatment, and the prevention of antisocial or delinquent behavior) are linked to increased school readiness outcomes. However, when considering the effect of home-based intervention on these, it is important to note the lack of longitudinal research findings to support the speculation that these outcomes may be affected in lasting ways by HV programs.

School readiness/success. The circumstances surrounding the birth and first few years of a child's life have the potential to significantly impact the child's development, and as such may affect the child's ability to begin school with the appropriate skills and behaviors included within the construct of school readiness. As success in school "can reduce the risk of involvement in risk behaviors that can compromise all forms of wellness" (Hawkins, 1997, p. 278), promoting services and environments supportive to children's academic success is a critical factor. In order to grasp the complexity of variables that influence school readiness and success, it is helpful to examine the above dimensions as they are influenced by the child's health, family environment, quality of early childhood care and education, school transitions, and community factors.

Studies indicate that children raised by both parents in a stable, positive, and caring environment benefit over those from chaotic and negative environments; the provision of financial support from an absent parent also has been linked to promoting school success (Emig, 2000). Given that "both academic failure and low commitment to schooling increase risk for later substance abuse, delinquency, school dropout, teen pregnancy, and violence" (Hawkins, 1997, p. 280), encouraging parents to adopt and model positive attitudes and practices around school success and commitment is a laudable goal. In particular, access to a print-rich environment at home predicts reading level at kindergarten and first grade. Beyond the availability of written text, opportunities to experience language, literacy, concepts of shapes and numbers, and the like through conversations, games, and encouragement all contribute to the academic indicator of "significant early experience" as defined by Phillips and Love (1997).

Ensuring children have access to community resources as early as possible maximizes the potential efficacy outside resources might have. Interagency communication between preschools and kindergartens increases the teachers' abilities to prepare students for any up-coming demands. Here again, parent-school contact and collaboration should ensure that children are supported at home and in the classroom (Emig, 2000). Each HV program should consider the needs and resources available within the community as they design and implement their service delivery model. Home visitors can serve as guides and resources in initiating relationships between schools and families. They also serve as positive role models for children and can demonstrate positive attitudes and behaviors around academic priorities. Beyond the children, parents can also look to home visitors to teach and support parents in establishing positive practices around schooling within the home.

Prevention of Antisocial/Delinquent Behavior

Like most things, antisocial and delinquent behavior is most glaring in outrageous quantities; however, the roots and most preliminary signs of a developing negative behavior pattern can be seen in some children's behavior as early as 3 years of age. Antisocial behavior includes a range of behavior from aggressive to withdrawn, instances of which are common in early childhood. It is when these "problem behaviors" have an extended duration, or an intensity that falls outside the purview appropriate for a given developmental stage, that a precursory pattern of antisocial or externalized behavior may rouse concern.

Often, children with behavior problems are placed together in remedial groups, which increases their exposure to negative peer influences and rejection by prosocial peers. Should parents respond to their child's antisocial or early delinquency with harshness or–even worse–violence, these children are even more likely to continue down a path of antisocial and negative behavior (Olds, Hill, & Rumsey, 1998).

Home visitation has proven a useful and effective intervention model in reducing the rate of juvenile delinquency rates (Olds et al., 1998). In a review of 18 HV programs and their effect on juvenile delinquency prevention, all 18 had some effect on risk factors contributing to delinquency, and/or rates of criminal activity or delinquency by the children when they entered adolescence (Sherman et al., 1998). However, when parental risk outcomes (such as maternal mental health and domestic violence) are evaluated in a randomized trial design, no significant overall program effects arise (Duggan, Fuddy et al., 2004).

NONTRADITIONAL OUTCOME VARIABLES: PROMOTING HEALTHY DEVELOPMENT

Healthy Families America (e.g., Daro & Harding, 1999) has three stated goals: to promote positive parenting, to encourage child health and development, and to prevent child abuse and neglect. Traditionally, the HV literature has focused primarily on the reduction of risk or mitigating the negative impact of risk factors through educational and other intervention. We draw on the resilience literature to examine several issues: how do we conceptualize a "healthy" person and family? What do we mean by wellness and well-being? We propose that HV programs consider measuring the following nontraditional outcomes: use of informal supports or community involvement and connection, maternal life course, parents' self-competence/confidence, and positive development.

Use of Informal Supports/Community Involvement and Connection

The proverb "it takes a village to raise a child" is most easily seen in American families by the connectedness of that family to the network of resources and supports that are available. Parents rely on family, neighbors, professionals, media and friends to resolve questions and problems on a range of topics that arise in parenting. Social support can increase parental capacities to care for children as well as buffer or protect the parent from negative consequences of a stressful event by providing specific resources for coping with stress. Those families that are isolated from these supports may struggle to find solutions to even the simplest problems that increase the risk to young children. HV is based on the premise that families benefit from the referral of issues and concerns to the appropriate support or resource. Some problems facing families with young children require support and resources that are not limited to single events, but rather to a lasting need best satiated by membership to a caring community (e.g., support groups, neighborhood communities, and continuing education opportunities).

Families at increased risk for neglect and maltreatment are often characterized as socially isolated which, as Thompson (1995) points out, is misleading in its incompleteness. Families at risk for neglect and maltreatment are often isolated from formal and informal social networks and resources that contribute a positive influence on the functioning of the family. Social support interventions must seek to integrate both natural and formal helpers into families' networks of support, not just promoting increases in volume or frequency, but in the constructive quality of supportive contact (Thompson & Ontai, 2000). Although recent randomized trials of one Healthy Start program indicate that paraprofessional home visitors may not be attuned to harmful parenting practices even in the highest-risk families and may subsequently fail to seek available community support (Duggan, McFarlane et al., 2004), HV is a likely formal service model that can accomplish the task of connecting families to individuals and communities that stand to support positive child development outcomes.

Along with an endorsement of HV to increase utilization of both formal and informal supports should come a caution: a formal service provider, like a home visitor, will only be successful in connecting parents to other resources if the natural sources of support already in place within the family will continue to support parents after HV has ended (Thompson & Ontai, 2000). This caution is based on the realization that HV will not serve as a cure-all for any family, that solutions to problems that face families with young children are most readily overcome by families who have formed a connection to a supportive community.

Data from HV models on social support and service utilization are limited. In a brief article summarizing a few benefits and challenges to the Healthy Families America model, McCurdy (2000) points out that HFA programs supported the increased use of preventive health care. However, there is no mention of the benefits derived from less formal sources of support and service utilization. Research to date has viewed social support and service utilization as two separate components of a family's resource network, and little evidence exists to support the effects HV may have on the use of informal supports or community involvement and connection.

Although data are scant regarding changes in parental social support, maternal social support is mentioned in the HV literature with some regularity. In particular, there is evidence to suggest that HV provides a degree of needed social support to mothers who report feeling isolated prior to their participation in HV programs (McCurdy, 2000). The efficacy of home visitors' efforts to connect families with additional supports is dependent on how many natural supports are available to the family (Thompson & Ontai, 2000). This includes family, friends and neighborhood resources preexisting to the home visitor's efforts. In summary, although few data exist to support the notion that HV may be the ideal model to increase a family's connectedness to a resource network within the community, the literature on the importance of these relationships is clear. Families at the greatest risk stand to benefit the most from changes toward supportive relationships and a sense of membership in an encouraging community.

Maternal Life Course

Olds et al. (1998) write that "[a] mother's personal development and lifestyle choices influence whether her child will develop antisocial behavior" (p. 3). Clearly these effects go beyond the purview of future antisocial behavior. Maternal life course can impact her children's physical and emotional well-being through the character of the environment in which the child will develop. Maternal life course is generally defined by a collection of events that mothers experience and choices that mothers make about the course they follow in life. Despite some variability, common elements include birth spacing of subsequent children, employment status, time on welfare and other public support, number of sexual partners, level of substance use, change in education level, and number of arrests (Olds et al., 1999). Each of these variables may be influenced by HV, depending on the focus of the program and the needs of the family.

Despite some varying program effects on maternal life course, there is evidence to suggest that HV is suited to encouraging mothers to make decisions that will improve their children's development as well. Home visitors are in a position to refer mothers to a variety of resources to support their achievement of personal goals (including the pursuit of education, changes in employment, or changes in health behaviors) and to encourage them to make these changes lasting ones that will extend beyond the duration of the HV.

Parents' Self-Competence/Confidence

Home visitation programs are often designed to impact parents' self-competence and self-confidence, as these constructs set the emotional stage for interactions between parent and child. Ensuring that parents have the knowledge to create appropriate and safe environments for their children is one of the many strategies used to promote not only positive parenting, but also a sense within the parents that they are capable of parenting their children well. For parents who have no positive parental model to follow and/or are isolated from both formal and informal sources of support, HV may be the best way to support the necessary skills and confidence to care for their children.

Nearly all types of HV include, at a minimum, situations in which the home visitor models developmentally appropriate behavior and activities for the parents to engage in with their children. It is also typical for home visitors to praise parents for their positive parenting and changes in interactions with their children, thus providing feedback to the parents and acting as a source of confidence building. Some studies report that programs that focus on parents' knowledge of and confidence in their ability to carry out developmentally appropriate interactions with their children are more likely to create developmentally stimulating environments for their children (Tracy, 2000). For the most part, however, studies rarely examine self-confidence and self-competence as stand-alone outcomes of HV. This may be because both constructs are highly subjective and somewhat difficult to measure. It may also be that HV programs are often designed to address the most pressing outcomes (e.g., health or maltreatment), rather than the mechanisms for the process of change (e.g., parent self-competence).

Positive Development

Resilience. Resilience is defined by Luthar and Cicchetti (2000) as "a dynamic process wherein individuals display positive adaptation despite experiences of significant adversity or trauma" (p. 858). For those children most at risk, or who face adversity in the home or at school, measures of resilience are helpful in understanding individuals' vulnerability and the protective factors that modify the child's experience of difficult events and enable them to adapt positively. Positive adaptation to adversity is comprised of the child's ability to continue to meet normative or developmentally appropriate tasks despite exposure to adverse or challenging events. The ability to meet these socially expected developmental landmarks is also a component of social competence, and in this way both competence and resilience are measures of adaptive behavior (Luthar & Cicchetti, 2000).

Resilience can easily be influenced by the presence of a home visitor in the family, as protective factors include the presence of a single positive relationship with an adult. Children at highest risk stand to benefit most from having a relationship with a trained home visitor. These visitors are in the position to negotiate changes in parenting and parent-child interactions, to support connections between the community and the child, to provide any specific service the individual child needs, and to encourage the family to persevere in the face of adversity.

Child/family wellness. It is relatively common to come across the term "wellness" when reading through the HV literature. Nearly all programs include a goal of improving or promoting children's wellness or well-being. Unfortunately, these terms are vague and ill-defined. For the purpose of HV, it is perhaps best to adopt a definition of "well-being" that is dominant in the psychological and social intervention literature. This definition of wellness is, in fact, a cluster of indicators on each of which a child can demonstrate a high or low ranking. These generally break down into the following dimensions: health, education, economic security, population, family and neighborhood, social development, and problem behavior (Brown, 1997).

In their meta-analysis of programs for the promotion of family wellness and the prevention of child maltreatment, MacLeod and Nelson (2000) defined wellness as "more than the absence of discord; it is the presence of supportive, affectionate and gratifying parent-child relationships and a stimulating home environment that is conducive to positive child development" (p. 1129).

RECOMMENDATIONS
FOR FUTURE PRACTICE, RESEARCH, AND EVALUATION

This review of home visiting outcomes underscores that some positive effects on children and families have been documented but that continued success will depend in large part on better documentation of impact. HV programs emerged from a focus on strengthening families, and that orientation continues to guide the outcomes of interest. We have attempted to call attention to additional aspects of healthy development that HV interventions theoretically may affect, such as connection to community, positive parenting, resilience, and wellness. The original focus on strengthening families has not yet translated into many measurable outcomes in this area, but they hold promise for future work.

Beyond documentation of the outcomes themselves, this review raises larger issues for HV models. First, it is important that programs recognize that the broad array of outcomes we have reviewed is just that–a *broad* array that may exceed the scope of an individual program. Programs should identify and prioritize those developmental outcomes that can logically be affected by their intervention. Second, such a prioritization requires that programs have clear ideas about the goals they are trying to accomplish and the means by which they can document success. What are the assumptions about preventing negative outcomes that guide an intervention–lack of parenting knowledge? Stress and poor coping skills? Only by identifying the pathways to prevention can programs specify what success should look like or how to train staff to capture these specific program effects. Third, clarifying goals and specifying outcomes for HV programs should occur in the larger community and service context. Fourth, the research reviewed in this paper highlights the importance of process, not just outcome. Successful interventions have the flexibility to respond to local context but retain the core elements of prevention theory and design.

Finally, we return to the fundamental issue of child development and strengthening families. HV models are guided by the assumption that parents are the best caregivers for their children, but that some parents may need knowledge, skills, and support in order to reach their parenting potential. Home visiting programs represent a promising–but still largely untested and undocumented–strategy for strengthening parents and communities and fostering positive developmental outcomes for children.

REFERENCES

Brown, B. V. (1997). Indicators of children's well-being: A review of the current indicators based on data from the federal statistical system. In R. M. Hauser, B. V. Brown, & W. R. Prosser (Eds.), *Indicators of children's well-being* (pp. 3-35). New York: Russell Sage Foundation.

Chaffin, M. (2004). Is it time to rethink Health Start/Healthy Families? *Child Abuse and Neglect, 28,* 589-595.

Chaffin, M., Bonner, B. L., & Hill, R. F. (2001). Family preservation and family support programs: Child maltreatment outcomes across client risk levels and program types. *Child Abuse and Neglect, 25,* 1269-1289.

Daro, D. A., & Harding, H. A. (1999). Healthy Families America: Using research to enhance practice. *Future of Children, 9,* 152–176.

Duggan, A., Fuddy, L., Burrell, L., Higman, S. M., McFarlane, E., Windham, A. et al. (2004). Randomized trial of a statewide home visiting program: Impact in reducing parental risk factors. *Child Abuse and Neglect, 28*, 623-643.

Duggan, A., McFarlane, E., Fuddy, L., Burrell, L., Higman, S. M., Windham, A. et al. (2004). Randomized trial of a statewide home visiting program: Impact in preventing child abuse and neglect. *Child Abuse and Neglect, 28*, 597-622.

Eckenrode, J. (2000). What works in nurse home visiting programs. In M. P. Kluger, G. Alexander, & P. A. Curtis (Eds.), *What works in child welfare* (pp. 35-43). Washington, DC: CWLA Press.

Eckenrode, J., Ganzel, B., Henderson, C. R., Jr., Smith, E., Olds, D., Powers, J. et al. (2000). Preventing child abuse and neglect with a program of nurse home visitation. *Journal of the American Medical Association, 284*, 1385-1391.

Emig, C. (2001). *School readiness: Helping communities get children ready for school and schools ready for children* (Research Brief). Washington, DC: Child Trends.

Furstenberg, F. F., & Hughes, M. E. (1997). The influence of neighborhoods on children's development: A theoretical perspective and a research agenda. In J. Brooks Gunn, G. J. Duncan, & J. L. Aber (Eds.), *Neighborhood poverty: Policy implications in studying neighborhoods* (Vol. 2, pp. 23-47). New York: Russell Sage Foundation.

Galano, J., Credle, W., Perry, D., Berg, S. W., Huntington, L., & Stief, E. (2001). Developing and sustaining a successful community prevention initiative: The Hampton Healthy Families Partnership. *The Journal of Primary Prevention, 21*, 495-509.

Garbarino, J., & Kostelny, K. (1994). Neighborhood-based programs. In G. B. Melton & F. D. Barry (Eds.), *Protecting children from abuse and neglect* (pp. 304-352). New York: Guilford Press.

Geeraert, L., Van den Noortgate, W., Grietens, H., & Onghena, P. (2004). The effects of early prevention programs for families with young children at risk for physical child abuse and neglect: A meta-anlysis. *Child Maltreatment, 9*, 277-291.

Hawkins, J. D. (1997). Academic performance and school success: Sources and consequences. In R. P. Weissberg, T. P. Gullotta, R. L. Hampton, B. A. Ryan, & G. R. Adams (Eds.), *Enhancing children's wellness* (pp. 278-305). Thousand Oaks, CA: Sage Publications.

Hawkins, J. D., Herrenkohl, T., Farrington, D. P., Brewer, D., Catalano, R. F., & Harachi, T. W. (1997). A review of predictors of youth violence. In R. Loeber & D. P. Farrington (Eds.), *Serious and violent juvenile offenders* (pp. 106-146). Thousand Oaks, CA: Sage Publications.

Korfmacher, J., Kitzman, H., & Olds, D. (1998). Intervention processes as predictors of outcomes in a preventive home-visitation program. *Journal of Community Psychology, 26*, 49-64.

Layzer, J. I., Goodson, B. D., Berstein, L., & Price, C. (2001). *National evaluation of Family Support Programs, Final report volume A: The meta-analysis.* Report prepared for the Department of Health and Human Services, Washington DC.

Leventhal, J. M. (2001). The prevention of child abuse and neglect: Successfully out of the blocks. *Child Abuse and Neglect, 25*, 431-439.

Leventhal, J. M., Garber, R. B., & Brady, C. A. (1989). Identification during the postpartum period of infants who are at high risk of child maltreatment. *Journal of Pediatrics, 114*, 481-487.

Luthar, S. S., & Cicchetti, D. (2000). The construct of resilience: Implications for interventions and social policies. *Development and Psychopathology, 12*, 857-885.

MacLeod, J., & Nelson, G. (2000). Programs for the promotion of family wellness and the prevention of child maltreatment. *Child Abuse and Neglect, 24*, 1127-1149.

McCurdy, K. (2000). What works in nonmedical home visiting: Healthy Families America. In M. P. Kluger, G. Alexander, & P. A. Curtis (Eds.), *What works in child welfare* (pp. 45-55). Washington, DC: CWLA Press.

McCurdy, K., & Daro, D. (2001). Parent involvement in family support programs: An integrated theory. *Family Relations, 50*, 113-121.

Melton, G. B., & Barry, F. D. (1994). Neighbors helping neighbors: The vision of the U.S. Advisory Board on Child Abuse and Neglect. In G. B. Melton & F. D. Barry (Eds.), *Protecting children from abuse and neglect* (pp. 1-13). New York: Guilford Press.

Nation, M., Crusto, C., Wandersman, A., Kumpfer, K. L., Seybolt, D., Morrisey-Kane, E. et al. (2003). What works in prevention: Principles of effective prevention programs. *American Psychologist, 58*, 449-456.

Olds, D., Henderson, C. R., Jr., Kitzman, H. J., Eckenrode, J. J., Cole, R. E., & Tatelbaum, R. C. (1999). Prenatal and infancy home visitation by nurses: Recent findings. *Future of Children, 9*, 45-65.

Olds, D., Hill, P., & Rumsey, E. (1998). *Prenatal and early childhood nurse home visitation.* Washington, DC: Office of Juvenile Justice and Delinquency Prevention.

Olds, D., & Kitzman, H. (1990). Can home visitation improve the health of women and children at environmental risk? *Pediatrics, 86*, 108-116.

Phillips, D. A., & Love, J. M. (1997). Indicators for school readiness, schooling, and child care in early to middle childhood. In R. M. Hauser, B. V. Brown, & W. R. Prosser (Eds.), *Indicators of children's well-being* (pp. 125-151). New York: Russell Sage Foundation.

Prilleltensky, I., & Nelson, G. (2000). Promoting child and family wellness: Priorities for psychological and social interventions. *Journal of Community & Applied Social Psychology, 10*, 85-105.

Reppucci, N. D., Britner, P. A., & Woolard, J. L. (1997). *Preventing child abuse and neglect through parent education.* Baltimore, MD: Paul H. Brookes Publishing Company.

Sampson, R. J., & Morenoff, J. D. (1997). Ecological perspective on the neighborhood context of urban poverty: Past and present. In J. Brooks Gunn, G. J. Duncan, & J. L. Aber (Eds.), *Neighborhood poverty: Policy implications in studying neighborhoods* (Vol. 2, pp. 1-22). New York: Russell Sage Foundation.

Sherman, L. W., Gottfredson, D. C., MacKenzie, D. L., Eck, J., Reuter, P., & Bushway, S. D. (1998). *Preventing crime: What works, what doesn't, what's promising. Research in brief.* Washington, DC: National Institute of Justice, U.S. Department of Justice.

Sweet, M. A., & Appelbaum, M. I. (2004). Is home visiting an effective strategy? A meta-analytic review of home visiting programs for families with young children. *Child Development, 75*, 1435-1456.

Thompson, R. A. (1995). *Preventing child maltreatment through social support.* Thousand Oaks, CA: Sage Publications.

Thompson, R. A., & Ontai, L. (2000). Striving to do what comes naturally: Social support, developmental psychopathology, and social policy. *Development and Psychopathology, 12,* 657-675.

Tracy, E. M. (2000). What works in family support services. In M. P. Kluger, G. Alexander, & P. A. Curtis (Eds.), *What works in child welfare* (pp. 3-9). Washington, DC: CWLA Press.

Wandersman, A., & Florin, P. (2003). Community interventions and effective prevention. *American Psychologist, 58,* 441-448.

Wolfe, D. A., Reppucci, N. D., & Hart, S. (1995). Child abuse prevention: Knowledge and priorities. *Journal of Clinical Child Psychology, 24,* 5-22.

doi:10.1300/J005v34n01_07

Healthy Families America® Effectiveness:
A Comprehensive Review of Outcomes

Kathryn Harding

Prevent Child Abuse America

Joseph Galano

College of William and Mary

Joanne Martin

Indiana University

Lee Huntington

Huntington & Associates

Cynthia J. Schellenbach

Oakland University

SUMMARY. This paper reviews 33 evaluations of Healthy Families America sites, with emphasis on 15 studies that include a control or comparison group. Outcome domains include child health and development, maternal life course, parenting, and child maltreatment. Parenting outcomes (e.g., parenting attitudes) show the most consistent positive impacts. Mixed results in other domains indicate the need for in-depth research to identify factors associated with better outcomes. Several

Address correspondence to: Kathryn Harding, Prevent Child Abuse America, 500 North Michigan Avenue, Suite 200, Chicago, IL 60611.

[Haworth co-indexing entry note]: "Healthy Families America® Effectiveness: A Comprehensive Review of Outcomes." Harding, Kathryn et al. Co-published simultaneously in *Journal of Prevention & Intervention in the Community* (The Haworth Press, Inc.) Vol. 34, No. 1/2, 2007, pp. 149-179; and: *The Healthy Families America® Initiative: Integrating Research, Theory and Practice* (ed: Joseph Galano) The Haworth Press, 2007, pp. 149-179. Single or multiple copies of this article are available for a fee from The Haworth Document Delivery Service [1-800-HAWORTH, 9:00 a.m. - 5:00 p.m. (EST). E-mail address: docdelivery@haworthpress.com].

factors that may contribute to differences in outcomes are discussed, including site implementation and quality, differences in family risk levels, and recent augmentations to program design. The paper also highlights two large-scale evaluations, one community-wide (Hampton, Virginia) and one statewide (Indiana), to illustrate exemplary evaluation approaches found in HFA research. Overall, HFA's continuing evolution has been positively impacted by researcher-practitioner partnerships.

doi:10.1300/J005v34n01_08 *[Article copies available for a fee from The Haworth Document Delivery Service: 1-800-HAWORTH. E-mail address: <docdelivery@ haworthpress.com> Website: <http://www.HaworthPress.com> © 2007 by The Haworth Press, Inc. All rights reserved.]*

KEYWORDS. Parenting, evaluation, prevention, child abuse

INTRODUCTION

Since the inception of Healthy Families America (HFA) in 1992, there has been a great demand for research on its effectiveness. This article provides a synthesis of HFA evaluation results to date (Part I) and an in-depth view of two large-scale evaluations to illustrate the strengths and complexities of HFA evaluation with regard to science and policymaking (Part II).

HFA provides home visits for new and expectant parents in over 400 sites around the country. The primary goals are to promote positive parenting, enhance child health and development, and prevent child abuse and neglect (Diaz, Oshana, & Harding, 2004). Rather than a strict replication model, HFA sites follow a set of critical elements that guide program implementation and services. This approach offers the advantage of research-based practice while permitting greater flexibility than standardized program protocols, allowing sites to tailor the details of program operations to suit local parameters. The HFA critical elements are based on research and practice in family support (e.g., Hawaii's Healthy Start Program), as well as theoretical work in the areas of attachment (Bowlby, 1969) and ecological models of child development (Bronfenbrenner, 1979). An important influence for HFA was Hawaii's Healthy Start Program, with its theoretical roots in Helfer's (1987) work emphasizing the need to "re-parent" the parent. For a detailed account of HFA's history and theoretical foundation, see Guterman, 2001).

An ongoing commitment to the integration of research and practice characterizes HFA at local, state, and national levels, with the vast majority of HFA sites (86%) engaging in some type of program evaluation (Prevent Child Abuse America [PCA America], 2001). Evaluations of all types share knowledge through a national network of researchers and practitioners (see Galano & Schellenbach, this volume). Despite this emphasis on research, synthesizing HFA evaluation results is challenging due to the same flexibility that makes the program attractive to and practical for local communities.

Flexibility in the model has given rise to tremendous variability in site implementation (Harding, Reid, Oshana, & Holton, 2004). HFA sites serve as few as 10 families at a time, or nearly 1,000, with an average of 110 current participants per program (Diaz et al., 2004). Sites determine the most appropriate target population (e.g., first-time parents or all births) and service initiation point (prenatal or at birth) depending on other services available in the community and local funding requirements. Sites select the curricula to use in home visits. Another variant is the risk level of enrolled families; some sites enroll predominantly those families at highest risk. Communities themselves also vary in risk (see Daro et al., this volume). Each of these differences may contribute to different patterns of results. Nevertheless, at this time, the field needs to take stock of what has been learned and what questions remain.

PART I: HFA EVALUATION OUTCOMES

In 1999, the David and Lucile Packard Foundation published a review of 17 HFA evaluations (Daro & Harding, 1999). Results suggested impacts in parent-child interaction and parenting capacity. The review included only two randomized controlled trials (RCTs), and three quasi-experimental studies. Subsequently, the number of evaluations with a control or comparison group has tripled, and many states have expanded their evaluation efforts as programs grow to statewide proportions.

Since 1992, the knowledge gained in nationally-affiliated[1] HFA sites has generated over 96 written reports on program outcomes (including eight published articles or books), representing 33 separate evaluations. This article reviews specific findings from these 33 evaluations, using the most recent report available for each evaluation.[2] In total, 288 Healthy Families sites in 22 states plus the District of Columbia participated in the evaluations reviewed, including 43 sites involved in RCTs. The appendix lists each study by research design. Additional details on the studies reviewed can be found at www.healthyfamiliesamerica.org.

This review emphasizes findings of more rigorous studies, but also includes outcome studies with quasi-experimental and non-experimental designs for two reasons. First, all but two of the RCTs conducted to date were begun in the earliest years of the HFA initiative and, not surprisingly, report numerous implementation problems. Many sites have made important improvements over the last decade, thereby limiting the applicability of these early studies for programs today. Second, the heterogeneity of HFA sites strongly cautions against over-generalization from one study to other sites. While RCTs provide the best assessment of program effectiveness, including multiple designs greatly increases the number of studies, offering some indication of the degree to which outcomes may generalize to other programs.

Eight of the studies are RCTs, with four using an intent-to-treat design (HI2, CA, AK, NY2). The eight quasi-experimental studies used a variety of strategies to form comparison groups, including one using multiple comparison communities (VA5), four using families meeting eligibility criteria but unserved due to program capacity (FL4,[3] HI3, MI) or program implementation date (WI), one using families enrolled in less intensive services (DC), and two using families who enrolled in HFA but terminated services very early (AZ) or declined services (FL3). The remaining studies (17) examine changes in program participants over time, compare program outcomes to established performance benchmarks, or provide cross-sectional results. Studies vary in scope from a single community to statewide.

Study outcomes are reviewed within four major domains: (a) child health and development (birth outcomes, breastfeeding, medical home, immunizations and well-baby visits, injuries, developmental screenings); (b) maternal life course (subsequent births, economic self-sufficiency, depression, substance use, and domestic violence); (c) parenting (attitudes, stress, behaviors, and parent-child interaction); and, (d) child maltreatment (official statistics and parent self-report). In this review, the term "significant" always indicates a probability of less than 5% ($p < .05$) unless otherwise noted.

Child Health and Development Indicators

HFA achieves child-health outcomes by linking families to a "medical home," that is, a regular health-care provider, and by encouraging compliance with recommended schedules of preventive health care such as prenatal visits, immunizations, and well-child visits. Staff also screen for developmental delays to identify and address problems as early as possible.

Birth outcomes/low birth weight (LBW). To impact birth outcomes, programs must enroll families early enough in pregnancy to reasonably expect change. Although not required by HFA, prenatal enrollment rates are increasing. In 2003, approximately 43% of all families were enrolled prenatally, compared to 36% in 2001 (Diaz et al., 2004).

Four studies (two RCTs) report comparisons on birth outcomes, all with positive findings. An RCT (VA2) found significantly fewer birth complications among home-visited families compared to controls (18% vs. 40% of infants with at least one birth complication). In a second RCT (NY2), mothers enrolled at least two months prior to giving birth had a significantly lower rate of LBW infants compared to their counterparts in the control group (3.3% vs. 8.3%), although the study found no differences in third trimester prenatal care, premature births, and need for neonatal intensive care. Other studies report reductions in LBW rates relative to community rates (FL3: 6.5% vs. 9.5% county-wide; DC: 3% vs. 10.6% in the program community). Two additional studies indicate that LBW rates met or exceeded program goals (NJ, VA4). These findings call for in-depth study, especially in light of generally poor outcomes across multiple home visiting models in this area (Gomby, 2005).

Breastfeeding. Although examined by only four of the studies reviewed, all report positive program impacts. Two RCTs (NY1, NY2) found a greater likelihood of breastfeeding among program mothers enrolled prenatally. In one RCT (NY2), home-visited mothers with two or more children were more significantly more likely to breastfeed than were their counterparts in the control group (50% vs. 40%); groups did not differ on the number of months of breastfeeding. In a second study (NY1), mothers who received prenatal home visits were twice as likely to report exclusive breastfeeding as were control and treatment group mothers who did not receive prenatal home visits (29% vs. 15% reported exclusive breastfeeding). A quasi-experimental study (WI) found that the program encouraged mothers enrolled within a few weeks of birth to breastfeed significantly longer (6.5 months vs. 3.6 months for comparison mothers). Finally, higher than expected rates of breastfeeding were found for teen mothers (MA: 63% compared to 55% of teen moms nationally).

Medical home. Sixteen studies (four RCTs), nine of them statewide, report outcomes on the percent of families linked to a medical care provider (AK, AZ, CA, FL3, FL4, HI2, IA, MD1, MD2, NY2, OR, TN, VA1, VA3, VA4, VT). Rates are consistently high (74% to 100%, averaging 94% across studies), yet none of the four RCTs reporting on this outcome found a significant difference between home-visited and control families (AK, CA, HI2, NY2). The different outcomes achieved by these methods are most likely due to the RCTs' inclusion of families assigned to the home visiting group despite their early termination of services (all four RCTs used an intent-to-treat design), while other studies count only outcomes achieved for families still enrolled at a given point of measurement. Results to date suggest that while families in HFA are consistently linked with medical providers, there is no rigorous evidence of program impacts on this outcome. Still, improved local statistics on health-care coverage for high-risk families would better assist programs in gauging their results relative to community-wide rates.

Immunization rates/well-baby visits. Twenty-eight evaluations report on one or both of these outcomes. None of the six RCTs examining immunization rates found program benefits (AK, CA, HI1, HI2, NY1, NY2). Two RCTs report significant positive impacts on number of well-child visits (CA, VA2), while two others found no program impact (HI1, HI2). A quasi-experimental study (WI) found significantly higher scores among Healthy Families participants on a combined measure of well-visits and immunization status. Other studies report higher immunization rates than local population rates (AZ, CT, GA, FL1, FL4, NJ, VA2, VA4), and the average rate of 87% across studies compares favorably to a national rate of 72% of children aged 19 to 35 months in households below the poverty level in 2001 (National Center for Health Statistics, 2004). However, as with findings on medical home above, these results provide no rigorous evidence for impacts on immunizations, and mixed findings on well-child visits.

Child development screening. The Ages & Stages Questionnaire (ASQ; Bricker & Squires, 1999) is widely used in HFA programs to screen for possible delays. Thirteen evaluations (AK, AZ, DC, FL1, FL2, FL3, FL4, MA, MD1, NJ, TN, VA1, VA4) report child development screening rates. The percentage of children screened ranges from around 50% to 100% (averaging 75% across studies). These findings reflect some challenges in completing screenings in many sites, most likely related to the challenge of engaging families.

Cognitive development. HFA focuses on improving parent knowledge of child development and screening for possible delays rather than direct interventions with children to enhance cognitive development; there is increasing evidence that cognitive impacts require intensive, direct intervention with children, such as enriched day care (Gomby, 2005; Nelson, Westhues, & MacLeod, 2003). Even so, five RCTs included developmental assessments. Two studies found significantly higher performance among home-visited children compared to controls. One (CA) found positive impacts at 1 and 2 years on the Bayley Scales of Infant Development

(Bayley, 1993), however, there was no difference at 3 years using the Stanford-Binet Intelligence Test (Thorndike, Hagen, & Sattler, 1986). Another study (AK) found evidence of positive impacts on cognitive development at 2 years on the Bayley Scales. The other RCTs (VA2, HI1, HI2) found no group differences at 1 year, or at 2 years (HI2). In addition, two RCTs (GA, NY1) and two comparison group studies (FL3, MI) report higher scores on the ASQ (primarily a screening tool) for home-visited vs. comparison children (NY1: only boys showed significant benefits). Because programs differ in their approach to enhancing child development, closer examination of program goals (e.g., school readiness vs. other outcomes), curricula, and involvement of home-visited children in enriched day-care settings such as Early Head Start may help to explain mixed results.

Summary of child health and development outcomes. This area shows several benefits of HFA. Consistently positive impacts on birth outcomes and breastfeeding, although examined by relatively few studies, suggest promise in these challenging areas. Mixed results on rates of well-child visits also merit further attention. In contrast, rates of immunization and linkage to a primary care provider, while consistently high, received no support in numerous rigorous studies. Developmental screening rates vary widely across sites, indicating a need for in-depth study to understand the factors related to higher screening rates. Finally, a few studies find modest evidence of program benefits on cognitive development.

Maternal Life Course Indicators

The HFA model seeks to support parents in a variety of areas beyond the parenting role per se. Although HFA provides a comprehensive set of recommended topics for staff training, each program determines its own strategy to address these issues. For problems such as maternal depression and substance abuse, some sites link families to community services; others add professional staff to work with families directly or closely supervise home visitors. Here again, variability across sites in their intervention approach contributes to mixed results.

Subsequent births. Six studies have compared home-visited families to others on subsequent births, with few positive results. Only one of four RCTs found a positive effect, and this was limited to Anglo mothers only (CA: 28% vs. 55% repeat birthrate over 3 years). Two RCTs found no significant group differences at 1 year (GA) or 2 years (AK). A fourth RCT (NY2) found a *higher* rate of repeat pregnancy among home-visited mothers than controls at 1 year, although this impact was limited to one of the three study sites. A comparison group study found no difference at 1 year (FL3). Although not a controlled comparison, a repeat birthrate for teens of 9.4% was found in comparison to 35.9% citywide (VA2), a notable difference. Other than RCTs with an intent-to-treat design, rates for repeat births and repeat pregnancy are typically reported only for mothers who remain in the program for the designated measurement period, so results may be confounded by other factors that influence parents' decisions to continue services.

Economic self-sufficiency. Maternal education, employment, and receipt of public assistance are often examined in HFA evaluations. One RCT (NY1) found significant impacts on maternal education, with home-visited mothers more likely than controls to increase their educational level by 24 months post-partum (18% vs. 7%). In contrast, four intent-to-treat RCTs (AK, CA, HI2, NY2) report no positive impacts on several indicators of maternal education and employment, with the exception of school attendance at year 3 in one study (CA). Also, one negative impact was found on maternal employment (NY2: 41% home-visited vs. 48% control mothers employed at 1 year), however this was not a primary focus in the first year of services. While less rigorous studies have noted increases in employment rates or education (AZ, DC, FL4, MA, MD2, MU, NJ), this area requires stronger evidence.

Two studies in this review (both RCTs) reported on receipt of public assistance (NY1, NY2), finding no program impacts. However, a study conducted in Arizona prior to welfare reform (Holtzapple, 1998), found that the percent of families on public assistance was lower among Healthy Families participants (46%) than comparison families (54%), and also found significant reductions in days on public assistance for Healthy Families participants.

Social support. HFA home visitors provide social support to new parents in the short-term, and attempt to help them develop social networks for longer-term support. Parent interviews describe the value of support received from home visitors (e.g., MA), yet most studies examine only support from family and friends. Ten studies (including seven RCTs) found no program impacts (AK, CA, HI1, HI2, GA, MD, MU, NY1, VA2, WI) using the Maternal Social Support Index (MSSI; Pascoe, Ialongo, Horn, Reinhardt, & Perradatto, 1988), which measures support from family, friends, and neighbors. In contrast, three studies using measures that assess formal (i.e., organized support services) as well as informal support report positive impacts (DC, MA, NJ). Findings overall suggest that few programs impact social support, but measurement differences may have contributed to the pattern of results.

Depression. Mental health problems, largely depression, are common among HFA participants, estimated at 21% of all enrolled mothers, and exceeding 50% in one out of 10 sites (Diaz et al., 2004). Maternal depression or general mental health was measured in five RCTs, of which three report limited evidence of program impacts. In one (NY2), significantly fewer home-visited mothers met the cutoff for clinical depression on the Center for Epidemiological Studies-Depression scale (CES-D; Radloff, 1977) at 1 year (23% vs. 38% of controls), although this impact was limited to one of the three sites evaluated (the investigators note the use of a clinical psychologist as the supervisor in this site); there was no difference in total CES-D scores. In another RCT (CA), home-visited mothers showed a significantly greater decrease in depression than control mothers from intake to 2 years on the CES-D. Groups did not differ at year 3. In the third RCT (HI2), home-visited mothers showed better general mental health than controls in one of the three agencies. This study found no group differences on the CES-D. Two RCTs (AK, NY1) found no program impacts on depression. Mixed results are also found with other study designs: a comparison group study (DC) showed significant reduction of depression symptoms on the CES-D at 6 months and maintained at 12 months among home-visited families vs. no change for comparison families, and a statewide study (MA) found significant reduction in depression among their population of teen mothers, although rates of depression at follow-up remained very high. Another comparison study (FL3) found no impacts. Although limited, these results suggest some potential for benefits; shortening the duration of maternal depression in a child's earliest years could reduce child maltreatment risk. Further examination is needed to identify practice differences related to this outcome that may guide future program development.

Domestic violence. The prevalence of domestic violence is estimated at 14% of HFA families, with 10% of sites reporting a rate of 33% or more (Diaz et al., 2004). Three RCTs examined rates of domestic violence over time. Two studies found no group differences at 2 years (AK) or at annual follow-ups over 3 years (CA). A third RCT (HI2) found a reduction in physical assault only for "high dose" families (defined as successful completion or still active at 3 years, received at least 75% of expected visits, and no more than 3 months on creative outreach). Many HFA programs have begun to enhance staff training to better address domestic violence issues, however, research examining these efforts is just beginning.

Substance use. The prevalence of substance use problems in HFA families is estimated at 13% averaging across all sites, with rates of 40% or higher in 10% of sites (Diaz et al., 2004). Of four RCTs examining changes in substance use, two report no impacts (AK, CA). One RCT (HI2) found a significant reduction in maternal problem alcohol use but only for families receiving a high dose of services (defined above). Similarly limited impacts were found in another RCT (NY2): number of cigarettes smoked per day was significantly lower among home-visited mothers under 18, and illicit drug use was lower among home-visited mothers in one of the three study sites. No differences were found on the number of smokers or alcohol abuse scores. Finally, a comparison study (DC) found no positive group differences at 1 year, providing further confirmation of the challenges of addressing substance abuse issues.

Summary of maternal life course outcomes. Impacts on maternal depression were modest but consistent across three RCTs and two comparison group studies, suggesting an opportunity and need for further study. Support for other maternal life course outcomes is minimal, with a few noteworthy findings (e.g., repeat pregnancy in VA2) that warrant further examination. In particular, more information is needed to determine the comparability of maternal risk factors across evaluations and site practices in order to address them.

Parenting Indicators

Research suggests developmentally responsive caregiving results in more attached mothers less likely to injure, abuse, or neglect their children (Olds, Kitzman, Cole, & Robinson, 1997). HFA staff provide education, modeling, and other activities designed to enhance parent-child interaction and help parents develop appropriate expectations of their children.

Parenting attitudes. Ten studies assessed parenting attitudes, most using either the Child Abuse Potential (CAP; Milner, 1986) Inventory or the Adult Adolescent Parenting Inventory (AAPI; Bavolek, 1984). Three RCTs (GA, HI1, NY2) report that home-visited parents improved at a greater rate on one or both of these measures than control parents, although for one study (NY2) the overall difference was only a statistical trend ($p < .10$). The latter found significant improvements for three subgroups: teen parents, the least depressed parents, and those served by one of the three sites involved in the evaluation. One RCT (AK) and a comparison group study (WI) found no group differences on parenting attitudes; neither study assessed rate of change. Other studies report significant improvements in parenting attitudes (CT, MA, MU, NJ). These results suggest that HFA may hasten positive changes in parenting attitudes.

Parenting stress. Eight evaluations examined this outcome, all but one using the Parenting Stress Index (PSI; Abidin, 1995). One of five RCTs

(AK) found that home-visited parents were significantly less likely to score at or above the 90th percentile on the PSI than were control parents at 2 years (22% vs. 30%, $p < .05$); group differences on total scores reached only a trend level of significance ($p < .10$). Four RCTs (CA, GA, HI2, NY1) found no significant program impacts, although one (CA) reported a trend ($p < .10$) favoring the home-visited families. Other study designs provide little support. One statewide comparison study reported *higher* stress among long-term participants compared to those who terminated services before 6 months, as measured by a single item on a telephone survey (FL4), and another study (MA) found increased scores on two PSI subscales, although total scores did not change significantly. A notable exception is a statewide study (AZ) which demonstrated significant decreases in parenting stress from intake to 6 and 12 months post-enrollment. An earlier phase of this study (LeCroy, Ashford, Krysik, & Milligan, 1996) included a comparison group, and showed significant reductions in parenting stress for HFA participants from baseline to 6 months, while stress increased for comparison group parents over the same period. Overall, however, there is very little evidence of program impacts on parenting stress.

Home environment. The HOME Inventory (Home Observation Measurement of the Environment; Caldwell & Bradley, 1984), used in 11 of the studies reviewed, is completed by a trained observer to assess stimulation and interaction provided to a child in the home context. Results from the six RCTs are mixed. Two RCTs found no program impacts on the HOME at 1-, 2-, or 3-year assessments (CA, HI2), while four (AK, GA, HI1, VA2) yielded positive program impacts at 6 months (HI1), 1 year (GA, VA2), 2 years (AK), or both 1 and 2 years (VA2). In addition to total score, improvements were reported for subscales measuring parent-child interaction (VA2, GA, HI1) and developmental stimuli (GA).

Studies using other designs consistently report positive impacts on home environment. Two quasi-experimental studies found significantly higher scores (WI) or greater improvement (DC) for home-visited mothers vs. a comparison group at 1 year. Four studies (AZ, IN,[4] MI, NJ) that assessed pre-post changes on the HOME show significant improvement. Another statewide study (VA4) found that 96% of scores were within the normal range on the HOME. Despite somewhat mixed results of RCTs, there is considerable evidence of HFA's impact in this area.

Parent-child interaction. The NCAST Feeding and Teaching Scales (Barnard, 1978), used by eight studies in this review, require observation of a caregiver and child by a trained individual. Findings on parent-child interaction (PCI) are mixed. Two of the six RCTs (HI1, VA2) found positive program impacts on one or both NCAST measures. The Hampton study (VA2) found that scores increased from baseline to 2 years in the home-visited group, including total score and subscales of sensitivity, child clarity, and child responsiveness, while scores of the control group families decreased over the same time period. In another RCT (HI1), home-visited families showed significantly increased parent sensitivity at 6 months, and greater child responsiveness at 12 months, relative to control families. These results are consistent with findings on the HOME in the two studies, described above, in which greatest gains were seen in HOME subscales that measure PCI. In contrast, four RCTs (AK, HI2, CA, NY1) found no group differences on the NCAST scales. Other findings on the NCAST include a pre-post study (FL2) with significant increases on the Teaching Scale at 1 year. Also, a statewide study (VA4) found 94% of scores were within normal limits. Compared to findings on the HOME Inventory, results with the NCAST scales are weak.

Summary of parenting outcomes. In general, parenting outcomes are positive, with greatest impacts on parenting attitudes and home environment, including subscales of the HOME Inventory measuring parent-child interaction (PCI). PCI measured by the NCAST scales demonstrated mixed results in RCTs. Here again, results suggest the need for more research to understand site differences in family risk level, community characteristics, and other factors, and whether these differences can explain the pattern of results.

Child Maltreatment Indicators

The use of child maltreatment rates as a measure of program effectiveness is problematic for numerous reasons. Assessing impacts on child maltreatment is a challenging and expensive task. The research team working with the Nurse-Family Partnership, one of the few home visiting models to demonstrate statistically significant program impacts on official rates of child maltreatment, has argued convincingly against the use of official maltreatment cases as evidence of program effectiveness (Olds, Eckenrode, & Kitzman, 2005). First, many cases of child maltreatment are not reflected in official rates (Sedlak & Broadhurst, 1996). Also, the small number of official cases relative to the population as a whole requires very large samples to detect differences. Third, real differences may be obscured by surveillance bias (Olds, Henderson, Kitzman, & Cole, 1995). Perhaps most importantly, child maltreatment rates do not capture the continuum of potentially harmful parenting behaviors and discipline practices. Many occurrences of harmful parenting behaviors may precede an incident of substantiated child maltreatment. HFA programs strive to prevent all harmful parenting behaviors, but outcome measurement is often restricted to only the most severe end of the spectrum. The above problems notwithstanding, 25 studies in this review assess child maltreatment rates.

Parent reports of child maltreatment avoid many of the limitations of official maltreatment rates, and despite the potential social desirability bias, parent reports have been found to identify more cases of maltreatment than official statistics (English, 1998). Four studies include the Conflict Tactics Scale-Parent Child version (CTS-PC; Straus, Hamby, Bonney-McCoy, & Sugarman, 1996), a self-report measure that includes neglect, psychological aggression, and a range of abusive behaviors from mild to severe physical assault.

Self-report child maltreatment outcomes. Four RCTs measured self-reported child maltreatment (AK, CA, HI2, NY2), all using an intent-to-treat design. The studies followed participants for 2 (AK) or 3 years (CA, HI2, NY2). Study findings are presented in detail below.

The earliest study of this group (HI2; conducted from 11/94 to 12/98, with 643 families) reports the least impact on self-reported child maltreatment. Only two program impacts were found across the 3-year study period using the CTS-PC. Self-reported neglect was significantly lower for home-visited mothers on a revised subscale and, in one of the three agencies, mothers were less likely to endorse a single item: "threatened to spank or hit child."

The second RCT (CA, conducted from 2/96 to 3/00, with 489 families) yielded slightly more positive outcomes. Mothers in HFA reported fewer incidents of psychological aggression at 2 and 3 years. Also at 3 years, home-visited mothers reported less use of corporal punishment.

More recent studies have yielded somewhat stronger outcomes. One RCT (AK, conducted from 1/00 to 7/03, with 316 families) found significantly lower rates of psychological aggression and mild physical assault across the 2-year study, but no difference in neglect or severe physical assault. Another RCT (NY2, begun in 2000 with over 1,000 study participants) has produced the most positive results to date, according to a report of first-year findings. Despite the brief time frame, the study identified positive program impacts on the CTS-PC, including subscales measuring psychological aggression, neglect, minor physical aggression, and severe/very severe physical abuse. Home-visited mothers used less psychological aggression overall, with significant subgroup impacts for the least depressed mothers and those free of domestic violence, consistent with other research (e.g., Eckenrode et al., 2000). Home-visited mothers also reported a lower prevalence of neglect. This impact was strongest for Latina mothers. Minor physical aggression was less frequent among home-visited mothers and, in one of the three study sites, was less prevalent among home-visited mothers. The greatest impacts for both prevalence and frequency of minor physical aggression were among home-visited families free of domestic violence. Finally, home-visited mothers reported less frequent severe or very severe abuse (collapsed into a single score) than control mothers, although the prevalence of mothers reporting severe or very severe abuse did not differ significantly by group.

Substantiated child maltreatment. Six RCTs (AK, HI1, HI2, VA2, GA, NY2) and four quasi-experimental studies (FL4, AZ, HI3, VA5) examined this outcome. In the first RCT of Hawaii's Healthy Start (HI1), a trend ($p < .10$) was found indicating fewer incidents of confirmed maltreatment among home-visited families (3.3%, all classified as "imminent harm") than among control families (6.8%, of which 62% were a type of neglect). The remaining five RCTs report no significant group differences on substantiated child maltreatment.

In contrast, three of four quasi-experimental studies report positive impacts on child maltreatment rates. A recent statewide study (FL4) found significantly lower rates of maltreatment among 753 families who completed the program[5] or received "high-fidelity" services[6] than for eligible families who could not be served due to program capacity. Further, most Healthy Families sites in Florida achieved the same or lower rate of maltreatment than non-served families in the same communities, with an overall rate of 4% for home-visited families vs. 5% for non-served families in the same communities, despite the fact that enrolled families are at greater risk than the general population. Another large study used hospitalization data (HI3) for over 3,000 families eligible for Hawaii Healthy Start services. Approximately half of the families enrolled in Healthy Start, and the remainder went unserved by the program due to capacity limitations. Because Oahu's medical system required that a child protection team evaluate every hospitalized child for potential child maltreatment, researchers were able to compare rates of child maltreatment hospitalizations between these two groups. Results showed that significantly fewer children were hospitalized for child maltreatment within the enrolled families compared to the unserved families (.27% vs. 1.70%, $p < .001$). A third study (VA5) found that reduction of citywide child maltreatment rates outpaced that of multiple comparison communities and regions with both higher and lower levels of risks and resources (see special section below).

Eight studies compared child maltreatment rates with a reference point such as county or community maltreatment rates. Seven of these studies (FL1, FL2, FL4, MA, NJ, OR, VA4) found apparently lower maltreatment rates among HFA participants (though not tested for statistical significance), with rates of 1% to 12%. For example, one study (VA4) reports a rate of 1.1% for home-visited children vs. an estimated rate of 4.7% for children in comparable low-income families nationwide (Federal Interagency Forum on Child and Family Statistics, 1997). Another (OR) yielded a rate of 1.3% for home-visited children aged 0-2 years vs. 2.5% for unserved children in the same counties aged 0-2 years. The remaining seven cross-sectional studies (IA, MD, MN, MU, VA1, VA3, VT) report maltreatment rates ranging from 0% to 8%, with all but two at 2% or less.

Summary of child maltreatment outcomes. Parent self-report measures of child maltreatment yielded modest program benefits, particularly for reductions in psychological aggression (three of four RCTs) and neglect (two of four RCTs). Reduction in official rates of maltreatment occurred in only one of six RCTs. However, three large quasi-experimental studies suggest substantial benefits of HFA in reducing child maltreatment. Also, many cross-sectional studies demonstrate lower maltreatment rates in home-visited families than expected, based on community rates.

PART II:
TAKING EVALUATION TO SCALE

Although a challenge for evaluation, HFA's flexibility to address diverse local needs made this an attractive model for citywide and even statewide adoption. In this section, we review two studies that take on the challenge of evaluating the effectiveness of large-scale programs. The first study measures community-wide benefits of a program that has scaled up to address the needs of an entire city, Hampton, Virginia. The second study examines a statewide program serving families in every county in Indiana.

Assessing Community-Wide Benefits:
Hampton, Virginia Benchmark Study

Improving health and well-being and reducing the incidence of child abuse and neglect for an entire community are the ultimate goals of many HFA programs. There are, however, many challenges associated with achieving and verifying these community-wide goals that have been well-documented in the prevention science and practice literatures. Given the central importance of developing and evaluating effective community-level preventive interventions that work in the natural environment, the Institute of Medicine (Mrazek & Haggerty, 1994) formally proposed the now well-accepted "Preventive Intervention Research Cycle" (PIRC), which has served as a guide for the field. Many funding sources and prevention researchers accept the model as the standard, and base program development and funding decisions on it. The PIRC model recommends a series of carefully planned steps including designing and testing preventive interventions in pilot studies, and extending the initial positive findings in larger field trials before moving to adoption and dissemination. A final step in the cycle is to conduct subsequent epidemiological studies to determine if the program actually resulted in reductions in the incidence of the targeted problem. The Hampton Healthy Families Partnership (HFP) is one of the few Healthy Families programs in operation long enough to complete the steps prescribed by the PIRC.

Since its inception in 1992, the Hampton HFP has focused on a single, overriding mission: to ensure that all Hampton children are born healthy and enter school ready to learn. These outcomes also contribute to the overarching city goal of making Hampton "the most livable city in Virginia," a designation awarded to the city by the National Civic League not once but twice in recent years. HFP is one of the first and most comprehensive programs in North America. A rigorous and comprehensive evaluation conducted by the Center for Public Policy Research of the Thomas Jefferson Program in Public Policy at the College of William and Mary (Galano & Huntington, 1999) spanned the first 6 years of HFP's operation, 1992-1998, and provided strong evidence of the program's impact.

The first component of HFP implemented was Healthy Start, a credentialed HFA home visitation program available to all families (first time and *"repeat"* mothers) at risk for child abuse and neglect. The randomized control evaluation found strong effects favoring program participants in the areas of reduced pregnancy risk status, birth complications, and repeat teen pregnancies, as well as better immunization coverage. There were moderate effects in the areas of parent-child interaction and the quality of the home environment. The child abuse and neglect findings were encouraging, but less conclusive because of practical and methodological limitations. Moreover, HFP in collaboration with the Hampton school system recently conducted an assessment of the school readiness of 56 Healthy Start graduates compared to all Hampton kindergarten students. The results suggest that these high-risk children were virtually indistinguishable from their general population peers (Hampton City Schools, 2004).

The second component of HFP, Healthy Community, was a comprehensive parent education program for all Hampton families with children. The Healthy Community component includes an extensive series of parent education classes, a "Welcome Baby" program (providing a home visit and a parent resource backpack for all new families in Hampton), Young Families Centers in all branches of the public libraries, and the Healthy Stages developmental newsletter. The evaluation of Healthy Community, using qualitative and quantitative approaches, suggested positive outcomes for all service areas, most notably the improved parenting skills and attitudes by participants of the parent education classes. There was also strong client satisfaction and community support for the partnership.

Based upon community support and the collective evidence of program effectiveness, a decision was made to bring the HFP's Healthy Start and Healthy Community programs to scale by 2003. This involved taking them from model demonstration programs reaching only a portion of those in need to a program available to all Hampton residents. At the same time, Partnership leaders commissioned a benchmark study (Galano & Huntington, 2002) to determine whether the initiative also proved effective at the community level, making the city a healthier place for Hampton's children and families. The study selected eight community-wide benchmarks reflecting the mission of the Partnership. The benchmarks were: prenatal care beginning in the first trimester, low birth weight babies, infant mortality, child abuse and neglect, childhood fatalities attributable to abuse and neglect, healthy birth index, assessment of reading/school readiness in kindergarten and first grade, and births to teens.

The study examined Hampton's performance and progress during a 17-year period between 1984 and 2000, and compared Hampton's performance to the Hampton Roads and Greater Richmond regions. Six Hampton Roads communities were also selected on the basis of an empirical analysis of 10 socio-demographic variables in all 17 Hampton Roads communities. Two communities were designated as peer communities, two as higher-resource, lower-risk communities, and two as lower-resource, higher-risk communities. This design allowed for comparisons that contrasted Hampton with two comparison regions, as well as with two similar communities, two with fewer risks and more resources, and two with more risks and fewer resources.

1. The study design employed two types of time-series analyses for each benchmark. The initial time-series analyses examined the period since the Partnership was initiated, including the preceding years (1991 and 1992) in order to establish a baseline. This analysis addressed change within communities and asked the question, did change occur during the intervention period?
2. The second analysis examined change between communities and asked, were there different rates of change between the communities during the intervention period?
3. The third analysis examined change pre- vs. post-intervention, and utilized an interrupted time-series design. The time frame for this analysis was more historical and compared an 8-year period preceding the initiation of HFP with an 8-year period beginning with the initiation of HFP. This analysis addressed the question, did changes prior to the intervention differ from changes since HFP's initiation, and were the trends for communities different?

Study results. While a complete presentation of the results of the study is beyond the scope of this summary, the overall findings of the Hampton Roads Benchmark Study (Galano & Huntington, 2002) were very positive. In almost all comparisons, Hampton compared favorably to the non-HFP communities. For brevity, this report focuses on two measures that best represent domains in which HFP can have an impact, infant mortality and child maltreatment. Hampton outperformed all of the comparison regions and communities on these measures.

Analyses of trends in infant mortality demonstrated that all of the communities experienced a reduction in infant mortality between 1991 and 2000. Although the R^2s (.66 for Hampton vs. .35 and .51 for Hampton Roads and Greater Richmond, respectively) were all significant, Hampton experienced the largest per year decline. Hampton's rate of change (−.99) indicated that the infant mortality rate fell by nearly one infant death per 1,000 infants per year, while the rates for Hampton Roads and Greater Richmond fell by .23 and .32 infant deaths per 1,000 per year, respectively. The differences between Hampton compared to Hampton Roads and Richmond were significant; the difference between the rates of change for Hampton Roads compared to Richmond was not.

The analyses of trends in founded cases of abuse and neglect for children born in Hampton, Hampton Roads, and Greater Richmond between 1991 and 2000 are summarized in Table 1 and indicate that Hampton experienced considerable success in reducing child abuse and neglect. The trend of declining child abuse and neglect was significant only for

TABLE 1. Child Maltreatment Rates 1991-2000 Change Within Communities

Communities	R2	Significance (*p*<)	Change (Rate per 1,000/Year)
Hampton	.72	.002	−.237
Hampton Roads	.28	.117	−.128
Greater Richmond	.084	.417	.07

Hampton ($R^2 = .72$, $p < .05$) and not for either Hampton Roads or Greater Richmond ($R^2 = .28$ and .08, respectively, $p > .05$). Indeed, Hampton's average rate over the decade was approximately 66% that of Hampton Roads (5.1 per 1,000 compared to 7.8 per 1,000, $p < .005$). Compared with Greater Richmond's rate, which actually increased during this time period (+.07 rate per 1,000/year) Hampton demonstrated a significant Community by Year interaction ($p < .005$).

Ecology and community context. It is also important to acknowledge that health occurs within a social, economic, and physical environment. As part of this study, the investigation examined whether Hampton's "social ecology" had become more or less conducive to health over the previous decade. That analysis confirmed that Hampton's encouraging performance occurred during a time when the Hampton community had experienced increased risk on a number of factors such as percent of children receiving TANF and unemployment rate This finding of progress in the face of growing risks and fewer resources suggests that the entire community may have become more resilient, resulting in less harm and healthier outcomes.

These findings are encouraging and support the original HFA vision of targeted interventions occurring within a broader context of universal, family-friendly services and supports. In Hampton, the targeted Healthy Start program took place within a larger context of serving all families. From the beginning, there was recognition that the at-risk label or the placement of the initiative under the traditional social service agency known for focusing on problems and troubled families would jeopardize the ability of the initiative to achieve widespread change (Galano et al., 2000). Providing services for all families through largely accepted institutions (e.g., libraries), and offering universal services was intended to build broad community support for the initiative. There is growing consensus that embedding prevention programs within the larger ecology can strengthen inter-organizational linkages, enhance grassroots and business participation, and strengthen community problem-solving (Miller & Shinn, 2005).

Policy implications. In 2004, the Senate Finance Committee of the Virginia General Assembly requested testimony designed to address whether the positive child and family health outcomes experienced by Hampton were associated with a reduction in treatment and rehabilitation costs. Figure 1 presents expenditures under Virginia's Comprehensive Services Act (CSA) for Hampton compared to Virginia between 1994 and 2004. This time frame corresponds to the initiation of HFP and HFP's going to scale. The significant difference between the trends in Hampton and the rest of the state is dramatic and clearly understood by citizens and policymakers alike. State officials across Virginia and in Hampton believe that HFP is one of the major reasons for this declining trend in Hampton. HFP, which began in 1992, has expanded rapidly, and it is both the *size* of the investment that Hampton has made in the Partnership and the *duration* of that investment in prevention that city leaders believe have resulted in the declining trends in CSA costs. In fact, a recent cost savings analysis documented that Hampton would have spent $11.2 million additional dollars if their CSA costs had risen at the same rate as the state of Virginia's. Partnership leaders believe that unless we are determined to eradicate child abuse, we can expect the cost of its associated remedial and therapeutic

FIGURE 1. Declining Comprehensive Services Act Expenditures for Hampton Compared to Increases for Virginia 1994-2004

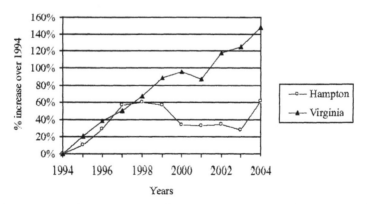

Note. Hampton: 1994–$2,561,087, 2004–$4,129,236; Virginia: 1994–$104,554,892, 2004–$259,323,434

services to go up endlessly. It is only by investing in prevention that the root causes of the problem will be addressed (Felitti et al., 1998).

Assessing Statewide Benefits:
Healthy Families Indiana HOME Study

The statewide evaluation of Healthy Families Indiana is one of a dozen statewide studies in this review. The substantial challenges of cost and logistics often limit state-level evaluation to cross-sectional studies with indicators of family well-being. In contrast, Healthy Families Indiana (HFI) uses more sophisticated longitudinal measures of progress which have been successfully implemented across the state. A statewide data management system permits detailed analyses of outcomes to inform ongoing program improvement.

Since 1994, HFI has offered home visiting services to families at higher risk of parenting difficulties. HFI encompasses 56 sites serving families in all 92 counties. The HFI Training and Technical Assistance Project at the Indiana University School of Nursing is conducting a longitudinal cohort study of 2,217 HFI families with a child born between January 1 and June 30, 1999. An advisory group of HFI state leaders guides all aspects of the evaluation to ensure relevance for practice and policy. While still in progress at this writing, the study has already demonstrated results on one of HFI's key objectives: parent-child interaction (Martin, Lang, & Ristow, 2003).

A statewide data system, the Home Visit Tracking Information System (HVTIS), forms the foundation of the HFI evaluation, ensuring uniform data collection on participant characteristics and HFI services provided, as well as outcome measures such as the HOME Inventory. HFI state leaders chose the HOME because it is designed to measure changes in parent-child interaction (PCI) over time. Three subscales measure PCI: Responsivity, Acceptance, and Involvement. Three additional subscales assess the physical environment of the home with regard to optimizing conditions for child development: Organization, Opportunities for Learning, and Variety of Materials.

At the onset of the study, use of the HOME was optional and only two-thirds of HFI sites had begun using it. Home visitors administered the HOME at least once to 816 families (49% of those enrolled at sites using the HOME, 37% of the total cohort). Only families who completed a second administration of the HOME during the target child's first year ($N = 421$) are included in this analysis. The HOME was typically administered when the baby was 2 to 3 months old, and again at about 6 months old. The average time between administrations was 3.3 months. Researchers compared families with two HOME administrations to those with only one or none to determine whether these groups were comparable. They found similar risk levels in the two groups on the Kempe Family Stress Checklist (FSC; median = 35 in both groups), but somewhat different patterns of risk factors. Mothers with two HOME scores were more likely to be Anglo, married, better educated, and have appropriate expectations of child development, but were more likely to experience low social support/depression and multiple stressors.

Study findings. HOME scores improved significantly between the first and second administrations, with mean scores of 30.17 and 34.02, respectively (paired $t = 14.45$, $p < .01$). In addition, five HOME subscales showed significant improvements over time (all but Acceptance).

This study did not have a comparison group to determine whether improvements on the HOME were due to HFI participation rather than maturation effects. The question of HFI's impact on HOME scores was, instead, addressed by examining service dosage and elapsed time in the program. Multiple regression analysis with two independent variables (number of weeks and number of home visits from the first to the second administration of the HOME) was significant ($F(2, 419) = 8.417$, $R^2 = .039$, $p < .001$), and showed a significant association for number of home visits and change in total score ($\beta = .224$, $p < .001$), while number of weeks was not associated with outcomes ($\beta = -.041$, $p = .546$). The number of home visits is significantly correlated with the number of weeks ($r = .710$, $p < .001$, 2-tailed). The individual effects may be lessened by this relationship. However, this does not mean the change in HOME scores is due to the passage of time. If number of weeks was removed from the regression, the significance of the number of home visits would likely improve. For every home visit, the HOME scale score increased by .22. This supports the expectation that participation in HFI home visiting contributes to improvement in HOME scale scores.

The study also examined the relationship between risk level and improvement on the HOME Inventory. Multiple regression analysis included four independent variables (number of weeks, number of home visits, mother's FSC score, and Time 1 HOME score), with Time 2 HOME score as the dependent variable. The overall model was significant ($F(4,416) = 79.175$, $R^2 = .432$, $p < .001$); significant predictors included Time 1 HOME score, number of home visits, and FSC score. This suggests that the relationship between the mother and baby at 6 months is a product of their earlier relationship, maternal risk factors, and the HFI intervention.

Lessons for statewide evaluations. The HFI evaluation demonstrates an approach to evaluation using data collected for multiple purposes within a common data system, making it economical while offering stronger evidence of effectiveness than broad cross-sectional indicators. Further, use of a standardized measure such as the HOME Inventory allows comparison with other studies. Limitations of this strategy include potential bias in using home visitors to collect data and quality issues typical of administrative data. However, in a statewide program, policymakers, funders, and administrators must find a balance between research concerns and practical considerations.

This study also demonstrates the impact that evaluation can have on program policy. When these data were collected, use of the HOME was optional. State policy now requires HFI sites to administer the HOME Inventory at regular intervals. Establishing the value of this tool for documenting program impacts contributed to higher compliance among sites and greater acceptance among home visitors of this additional responsibility.

DISCUSSION:
UNDERSTANDING MODEST SUCCESSES

Almost all of the 33 HFA evaluations reviewed are of field-based programs rather than demonstration sites. Although high on external validity, they are subject to real-world constraints such as budget cuts and midstream design modifications. Many sites struggle to maintain funding yet recognize the necessity of evaluation and the benefits of improving practice through research. As such, the authors feel a responsibility to go beyond pronouncements of program impact by striving to mine this rich data source for lessons to guide program development.

The studies reviewed demonstrated strongest outcomes in the parenting domain, consistent with other reviews of HFA sites (Daro & Harding, 1999) and home visiting in general (Gomby, 2005). This review also found support for an impact on child health, with the majority of more rigorous studies demonstrating at least one positive outcome. Developmental screening rates vary widely, reflecting the challenge of completing initial screenings; results on cognitive development, on the other hand, may indicate a greater potential for benefits in this area. Maternal life course outcomes yielded positive impacts in only a few studies, with the exception of reduction in maternal depression (or mental health issues) in five of eight studies. Parent self-report measures and very large population-based or quasi-experimental studies showed limited positive impacts on child maltreatment. Most RCTs found no impact on confirmed reports of maltreatment. Given the association between maternal risk factors of depression, substance abuse, and domestic violence with child maltreatment, and the prevalence of these factors among HFA participants at enrollment, it should not be surprising to find that child maltreatment rates were often unaffected.

The varying results of HFA mirror the variability of its implementation. Gomby, Culross, and Behrman (1999) raised the possibility that implementation differences might account for mixed outcomes in home visiting. The findings from the largest HFA implementation study to date[7] confirm that many program elements vary greatly from one site to the next (Harding et al., 2004). For example, while all sites offer weekly visits and long-term enrollment, actual intensity and duration of services vary widely. Sites even vary in how they interpret program goals and the strategies they use to achieve them. Further study is needed to understand the causes of implementation differences as well as the effect on outcomes.

Variability in HFA outcomes may also be an issue of quality. A key strategy for quality assurance in HFA is a credentialing process overseen by PCA America (see Holton & Harding; Friedman & Schreiber, this volume). Since 1997, HFA credentialing has provided a rigorous, standardized assessment of program quality using trained peer reviewers. Of the eight RCTs reviewed here, only two (AK, NY2) involved sites that completed HFA credentialing prior to the onset of the study. Without a standardized measure of quality, it is difficult to determine the extent to which quality differs across sites.

While implementation and quality issues are common obstacles to successful program replication, a hidden factor may be differences in family risk level. HFA and most comparable home visiting programs typically describe participants as "at-risk," with the general assumption that family risk level is comparable across sites. This is not the case in HFA. A multi-state study of HFA implementation (Harding et al., 2004) found that median family risk level was twice as high in some sites as in others (n = 56 sites in 5 states); 25% of study sites had a mean family risk score in the high-risk range. While there is some evidence that home visiting programs are more likely to yield significant outcomes with moderate-risk than high-risk families (Bugental et al., 2002), HFA sites are typically not willing or able to turn away higher-risk families. Instead, the field must continue to work toward the goal of effectively serving high-risk families. It would be wise for HFA evaluations to report information on baseline family risk as a potential moderator of program success. Further, sites that provide evidence of benefits for high-risk families would be of tremendous value to the prevention field as a whole.

The relationship between family risk factors and outcomes is complex. Risk factors such as domestic violence, depression, and substance abuse may be more closely associated with child maltreatment and have been shown to inhibit benefits in HFA (e.g., AK, NY2) and other home visiting models (e.g., Eckenrode et al., 2000). Differences in the prevalence of key risk factors in each study sample would be expected to influence the pattern of outcomes. Indeed, recent findings in New York State's RCT (DuMont, Mitchell-Herzfeld, Greene, Lee, & Rodriguez, 2006) show stronger impacts on child maltreatment for young, first-time mothers who enrolled during pregnancy, and for women with depressive symptoms and a low sense of mastery. These two subgroups benefited to a greater degree than the more heterogeneous sample that is characteristic of HFA. The study authors suggest that stronger outcomes in the NY study relative to other HFA evaluations may be due to NY's inclusion of prenatally-enrolled families, whereas some HFA evaluations include only post-natally enrolled families (e.g., San Diego). The degree to which target population characteristics impact outcomes is a central question in the ongoing effort to improve the effectiveness of home visitation.

Based upon our growing knowledge of risk factors, many programs have enhanced staff training and augmented services to help identify and address critical risk factors (e.g., Ammerman et al., this volume). The use of motivational interviewing, a tool to enhance motivation for change with challenging problems such as substance abuse (Miller & Rollnick, 1991), is increasing in HFA. Evaluators should assess and report the prevalence of major risk factors in the study sample, include detailed descriptions of program enhancements intended to address these risks, and conduct subgroup analyses to determine their influence on program impacts.

Research to date has identified challenges for home visiting and informed the development of important enhancements, yet few evaluations have provided a rigorous test of such innovations. One exception is a study by Bugental et al. (2002), an RCT of a home visiting program similar to HFA's model augmented with a cognitive retraining intervention component targeting parents' attributions for their infants' behavior. They found significant reductions in parent reports of child maltreatment at 1 year on the Conflict Tactics Scale. HFA's flexibility accommodates such innovations, and the national network of HFA sites and state leaders provides a conduit for diffusion. The steep learning curve of HFA's first decade has led to considerable program enhancement and some positive findings not evident in the earliest evaluations.

HFA evaluations have also improved in the past decade. Comprehensive home visiting programs like HFA are a challenge to implement (Gomby et al., 1999), and assessing implementation is critical to understanding and achieving results as well as replicating programs (Durlak, 1998). Increasingly, evaluation efforts provide guidance for program improvement, and help illuminate common problems across programs to inform national quality improvement efforts (Oshana, Harding, Friedman, & Holton, 2005). Over the history of HFA's development, despite little or no funding, many evaluators have formed long-term partnerships with local programs, representing an ideal of applied science. Moreover, through such partnerships, programs have continuously evolved to address needs identified by research. HFA stands as a model for integrating evaluation research and practice (see Galano & Schellenbach, this volume).

Evaluating the success of HFA is a continuous process, necessitated by the program's ongoing evolution. In order to strengthen programs, research must identify the key ingredients for prevention and associated contextual factors required for success (Guterman, 2001). This special issue illustrates the broad range of current research with HFA to achieve this goal. In particular, several researchers affiliated with the HFA network have begun to unravel the complex dynamics of family engagement and retention in voluntary preventive services (e.g., Ammerman et al., 2006; Daro et al., this volume; Daro, McCurdy, Falconnier, & Stojanovic, 2003; McGuigan, Katzev, & Pratt, 2003). As noted by Guterman (2001), a critical challenge for home visiting is the growing evidence that factors influencing participation rates are often cited as etiological factors in physical child abuse and neglect itself.

While there is a need to strategically strengthen home visiting programs, this review demonstrates that some Healthy Families programs achieve many of the hoped-for outcomes. A case in point, in January of 2006, Healthy Families New York (HFNY) achieved designation as a "proven program" by the RAND Corporation's Promising Programs Network. HFNY is only the second home visiting model to be awarded this distinction, determined by stringent criteria for research methodology and outcomes.[8] Positive findings to date may be considered indicators of what *can* be achieved by this model and replicated in other sites by gaining a better understanding of requisite practices.

To move the prevention field forward, researchers and funders must attend to both process and outcome measurement, so that study results tell us not only the outcomes achieved but why. Further, as recommended by Wandersman, Kloos, Linney, and Shinn (2005), research on HFA should include lessons from local sites and communities about effective adaptations of the basic HFA model (e.g., Ammerman et al., this volume; Krysik & LeCroy, this volume) and how to replicate such practices in other sites (Miller & Shinn, 2005). By examining the pathways from specific practices to outcomes we will understand why some sites succeed where others struggle, and we will strengthen our nationwide network of support for young families.

NOTES

1. To become affiliated with HFA and use the trademarked name "Healthy Families" as part of a program's name, sites must adhere to all of the HFA critical elements and agree to complete the HFA credentialing process following an initial implementation period. There are numerous sites based on the HFA model that are not affiliated. This review includes only evaluations of sites that are affiliated or were affiliated at the time the evaluation was conducted.

2. Multiple reports on a single evaluation were reviewed in a few cases when necessary to gain a comprehensive picture of evaluation methods and results.

3. This study included an additional comparison group of families who terminated services early in the program.

4. The Indiana study is presented in detail in the section on statewide evaluation.

5. Program completion was defined as on Level 4 for at least 3 months, home environment is stable and nurturing, child's growth and development are age appropriate, immunizations are up-to-date and the project and family agree to end services.

6. High fidelity was defined as enrolled at least 3 years, received at least 75% of expected visits, and on creative outreach less than 3 months.

7. Funded by the David and Lucile Packard Foundation and the Gerber Foundation, 1999-2003.

8. See http://www.promisingpractices.net/newsletters/news0601.asp.

REFERENCES

Abidin, R. R. (1995). *Parenting Stress Index administration manual* (3rd Ed.). Odessa, FL: Psychological Assessment Resources, Inc.

Ammerman, R. T., Stevens, J., Putnam, F. W., Altaye, M., Hulsmann, J. E., Lehmkuhl, H. D., Monroe, J. C., Gannon, T. A., & Van Ginkel, J. B. (2006). Predictors of early engagement in home visitation. *Journal of Family Violence, 21*(2), 105-115.

Barnard, K. E. (1978). Nursing Child Assessment Satellite Training Learning Resource Manual. Seattle: University of Washington.

Bavolek, S. J. (1984). *Handbook for the Adult-Adolescent Parenting Inventory*. Eau Claire, WI: Family Development Associates, Inc.

Bayley, N. (1993). *Bayley Scales of Infant Development* (2nd Ed.). New York: The Psychological Corporation.

Bowlby, J. (1969). *Attachment and loss: Vol. 1. Attachment*. New York: Basic Books.

Bricker, D., & Squires, J. (1999). *Ages and Stages Questionnaires (ASQ): A parent-completed child-monitoring system* (2nd ed.). Baltimore: Paul Brookes.

Bronfenbrenner, U. (1979). *The ecology of human development: Experiments by nature and design.* Cambridge, MA: Harvard University Press.

Bugental, D. B., Ellerson, P. C., Lin, E. K., Rainey, B., Kokotovic, A., & O'Hara, N. (2002). A cognitive approach to child abuse prevention. *Journal of Family Psychology, 16,* 243-258.

Caldwell, B., & Bradley, R. (1984). *Home observation for measurement of the environment.* Little Rock, AR: University of Arkansas.

Daro, D., & Harding, K. (1999). Healthy Families America: Using research to enhance practice. *The Future of Children, 9*(1), 152-176.

Daro, D., McCurdy, K., Falconnier, L., & Stojanovic, D. (2003). Sustaining new parents in home visitation services: Key participant and program factors. *Child Abuse and Neglect, 27,* 1101-1125.

Diaz, J., Oshana, D., & Harding, K. (2004). *Healthy Families America: 2003 profile of program sites.* Chicago: Prevent Child Abuse America.

DuMont, K., Mitchell-Herzfeld, S., Greene, R., Lee, E., Lowenfels, A., & Rodriguez, M. (2006). *Healthy Families New York (HFNY) randomized trial: Impacts on parenting after the first two years.* New York State Office of Children & Family Services. Retrieved July 19, 2006, from www.ocfs.state.ny.us/main/prevention/assets/HFNYRandomizedTrialWorkingPaper.pdf

Durlak, J. A. (1998). Why program implementation is important. *Journal of Prevention & Intervention in the Community, 17*(2), 5-18.

Eckenrode, J., Ganzel, B., Henderson, C. R., Smith, E., Olds, D., Powers, J. et al. (2000). Preventing child abuse and neglect with a program of nurse home visitation: The limiting effects of domestic violence. *Journal of the American Medical Association, 284*(11), 1385-1391.

English, D. J. (1998). The extent and consequences of child maltreatment. *The Future of Children, 8,* 39-53.

Federal Interagency Forum on Child and Family Statistics (1997). *America's children: Key national indicators of well-being.* Washington, DC: U.S. Government Printing Office.

Felitti, V. J., Anda, R. F., Nordenberg, D., Williamson, D. F., Spitz A. M., Edwards V. et al. (1998). Relationship of childhood abuse and household dysfunction to many of the leading causes of death in adults. The Adverse Childhood Experiences (ACE) Study. *American Journal of Preventive Medicine, 14,* 245-258.

Galano, J., Credle, W., Perry, D., Berg, S., Huntington, L., & Stief, E. (2000). Developing and sustaining a successful community prevention initiative: The Hampton Healthy Families Partnership. *Journal of Primary Prevention, 21,* 495-509.

Galano, J., & Huntington, L. (1999). *Evaluation of the Hampton, Virginia, Healthy Families Partnership: 1992-1998.* Center for Public Policy Research, The Thomas Jefferson Program in Public Policy, The College of William and Mary, Williamsburg, VA.

Galano, J., & Huntington, L. (2002). *FY 2002 Healthy Families Partnership Benchmark Study: Measuring community-wide impact.* Prepared by the Applied Social Psychology Research Institute, College of William and Mary, Williamsburg, VA.

Gomby, D. S. (2005). *Home Visitation in 2005: Outcomes for children and parents.* Invest in Kids Working Paper No. 7. Washington, DC: Committee for Economic

Development. Retrieved September 26, 2005, from www.ced.org/docs/report/ report_ivk_gomby_2005.pdf

Gomby, D. S., Culross, P. L., & Behrman, R. E. (1999). Home visiting: Recent program evaluations–Analysis and recommendations. *The Future of Children, 9*(1), 4-26.

Guterman, N. B. (2001). *Stopping child maltreatment before it starts.* Thousand Oaks, CA: Sage Publications, Inc.

Hampton City Schools (2004). *2004 report on school readiness.* Department of Psychological Services, Research and Evaluation, Hampton, VA.

Harding, K., Reid, R., Oshana, D., & Holton, J. (2004). *Initial results of the HFA implementation study.* Report to the David and Lucile Packard Foundation. Prevent Child Abuse America, Chicago.

Helfer, R. E. (1987). The developmental basis of child abuse and neglect: An epidemiological approach. In R. E. Helfer & R. S. Kempe (Eds.), *The battered child* (4th ed., pp. 60-80). Chicago: University of Chicago Press.

Holtzapple, E. (1998, July). *Evaluation of Arizona's Healthy Families pilot program.* Paper presented at Program Evaluation and Family Violence Research: An International Conference, Durham, NH.

LeCroy, C., Ashford, J., Krysik, J., & Milligan, K. (1996). *Healthy Families Arizona: Evaluation report for Tucson, Prescott, and Casa Grande sites, 1992-1994.* Phoenix: Arizona Department of Economic Security.

Martin, J., Lang, M., & Ristow, R. (2003). *HOME scale results from Healthy Families Indiana.* Report to Healthy Families Indiana Advisory Committee.

McGuigan, W. M., Katzev, A. R., & Pratt, C. C. (2003). Multi-level determinants of retention in a home-visiting child abuse prevention program. *Child Abuse and Neglect, 27*, 359-361.

Miller, R. L., & Shinn, M. (2005). Learning from communities: Overcoming difficulties in dissemination of prevention and promotion efforts. *American Journal of Community Psychology, 35*(3/4), 169-183.

Miller, W. R., & Rollnick, S. (1991). *Motivational interviewing: Preparing people to change addictive behavior.* New York: Guilford Press.

Milner, J. S. (1986). *The Child Abuse Potential Inventory: Manual.* Webster, NC: Psytech, Inc.

Mrazek, P. J., & Haggerty, R. J. (Eds.) (1994). *Reducing risks for mental disorders: Frontiers for preventive intervention research.* Institute of Medicine. Washington DC: National Academy Press.

National Center for Health Statistics (2004). *Health, United States, 2004 with chartbook on trends in the health of Americans.* Hyattsville, MD: U.S. Government Printing Office. Retrieved February 12, 2005 from http://www.cdc.gov/nchs/hus.htm

Nelson, G., Westhues, A., & MacLeod, J. (2003). A meta-analysis of longitudinal research on preschool programs for children. *Prevention & Treatment, 6*, 1-31.

Olds, D., Eckenrode, J., & Kitzman, H. (2005, March). Clarifying the impact of the Nurse-Family Partnership on child maltreatment: Response to Chaffin (2004) [Letter to the Editor]. *Child Abuse and Neglect, 29*, 229-234.

Olds, D., Henderson, C. R., Kitzman, H., & Cole, R. (1995). Effects of prenatal and infancy nurse home visitation on surveillance of child maltreatment. *Pediatrics, 95*, 365-372.

Olds, D., Kitzman, H., Cole, R., & Robinson, J. (1997). Theoretical foundations of a program of home visitation for pregnant women and parents of young children. *Journal of Community Psychology, 24,* 9-25.

Oshana, D., Harding, K., Friedman, L., & Holton, J. (2005, March). Rethinking Healthy Families: A continuous responsibility [Letter to the Editor]. *Child Abuse and Neglect, 29,* 219-228.

Pascoe, J., Ialongo, N., Horn, W., Reinhardt, M., & Perradatto, D. (1988). The reliability and validity of the Maternal Social Support Index. *Family Medicine, 20,* 271-276.

Prevent Child Abuse America (2001). *Healthy Families America–Annual profile of program sites: 2000.* Chicago.

Radloff, L. S. (1977). The CES-D scale: A self-report depression scale for research in the general population. *Applied Psychological Measurement, 1,* 395-401.

Sedlak, A. J., & Broadhurst, D. D. (1996). *The third national incidence study of child abuse and neglect.* Washington, DC: US Department of Health and Human Services.

Straus, M. A., Hamby, S. L., Bonney-McCoy, S., & Sugarman, D. B. (1996). The revised conflict tactics scales (CTS2). *Journal of Family Issues, 17,* 283-316.

Thorndike, R. L., Hagen, E. P., & Sattler, J. M. (1986). *Stanford-Binet Intelligence Test* (4th ed.). Chicago: Riverside Publishing Co.

Wandersman, A., Kloos, B., Linney, J. A., & Shinn, M. (2005). Science and community psychology: Enhancing the vitality of community research and action. *American Journal of Community Psychology, 35*(3/4), 105-106.

doi:10.1300/J005v34n01_08

APPENDIX: Evaluations

Code	Location/Scope	Design	Year of Report	Principal Investigator(s)
AK	Statewide (6 sites)	RCT	2005	Duggan, A.
AZ	Statewide (14 sites)	Mixed methods	2004	LeCroy, C.
CA	San Diego (1 site)	RCT	2002	Landsverk, J.
CT	Statewide (5 sites)	single group	2000	Black, T.
DC	1 site	Comparison	2005	Klagholz, D.
FL1	Pinellas County (3 sites)	single group	2001	Nelson, C.
FL2	Orange County (1 site)	single group	2001	Carnahan, S.
FL3	Jacksonville (1 site)	Comparison	2001	Edwards, C.
FL4	Statewide (42 sites)	Comparison	2005	Williams, J.
GA	8 sites	RCT	1999	Chambliss, J.
HI1	2 sites	RCT	1996	Daro, D.
HI2	6 sites	RCT	2004	Duggan, A.
HI3	6 sites	Comparison	2004	Breakey, G., Dew, B.
IA	Statewide (13 sites)	single group	2004	Iowa Department of Public Health
IN	Statewide (56 sites)	single group	2004	Martin, J.
MA	Statewide (22 sites)	single group	2005	Jacobs, F., Easterbrooks, M.A.
MD1	Statewide (13 sites)	single group	2002	Klagholz, D.
MD2	Montgomery Co. (1 site)	single group	2005	Klagholz, D.
MI	Oakland Co. (1 site)	Comparison	1999	Schellenbach, C.
MN	1 site	single group	1998	Chase, R.
MU*	OK, NV, WI (3 sites)	single group	1998	Harding, K., Daro, D.
NJ	Statewide (17 sites)	single group	2000	Dellano, D., Dundon, W.
NY1	New York City (1 site)	RCT	2004	Anisfeld, E.
NY2	3 sites	RCT	2005	Mitchel-Herzfeld, S.
OR	Statewide (15 sites)	single group	2001	Katzev, A.
TN	Statewide (8 sites)	single group	2002	Pope, B.
VA1	Alexandria (1 site)	single group	1996	Barrett, B.
VA2	Hampton (1 site)	RCT	1999	Galano, J.
VA3	Prince William (1 site)	single group	1998	Barrett, B.
VA4	Statewide (33 sites)	single group	2004	Galano, J.
VA5	Hampton (1 site)	Comparison	2002	Galano, J.
VT	Newport (1 site)	single group	2001	Vermont Department of Health
WI	Walworth Co. (1 site)	Comparison	1998	Keim, A.

*MU is used as the study code for a multi-state evaluation.

The Role of Community
in Facilitating Service Utilization

Deborah Daro
Chapin Hall Center for Children, University of Chicago

Karen McCurdy
Human Development and Family Studies, University of Rhode Island

Lydia Falconnier
School of Social Work, University of Illinois at Chicago

Carolyn Winje
Chapin Hall Center for Children, University of Chicago

Elizabeth Anisfeld
Best Beginnings, Columbia University College of Physicians & Surgeons, Department of Pediatrics

Aphra Katzev
Bates Family Study Center, Oregon State University

Ann Keim
Cooperative Extension, University of Wisconsin

Craig W. LeCroy
School of Social Work, University of Arizona

Address correspondence to: Deborah Daro, Research Fellow, The Chapin Hall Center for Children, 1313 East 60th Street, Chicago, IL 60637 (E-mail: daro-deborah@chmail.spc.uchicago.edu).

[Haworth co-indexing entry note]: "The Role of Community in Facilitating Service Utilization." Daro, Deborah et al. Co-published simultaneously in *Journal of Prevention & Intervention in the Community* (The Haworth Press, Inc.) Vol. 34. No.1/2, 2007, pp. 181-204; and: *The Healthy Families America® Initiative: Integrating Research, Theory and Practice* (ed: Joseph Galano) The Haworth Press, 2007, pp. 181-204. Single or multiple copies of this article are available for a fee from The Haworth Document Delivery Service [1-800-HAWORTH, 9:00 a.m. - 5:00 p.m. (EST). E-mail address: docdelivery@haworthpress.com].

William McGuigan

Human Development & Family Studies, Penn State University

Carnot Nelson

Department of Psychology, University of South Florida

SUMMARY. Guided by an integrated theory of parent participation, this study examines the role community characteristics play in influencing a parent's decision to use voluntary child abuse prevention programs. Multiple regression techniques were used to determine if different community characteristics, such as neighborhood distress and the community's ratio of caregivers to those in need of care, predict service utilization levels in a widely available home visiting program. Our findings suggest that certain community characteristics are significant predictors of the extent to which families utilize voluntary family supports over and above the proportion of variance explained by personal characteristics and program experiences. Contrary to our initial assumptions, however, new parents living in the most disorganized communities received more home visits than program participants living in more organized communities. The article concludes with recommendations on how community capacity building might be used to improve participant retention. doi:10.1300/J005v34n01_09 *[Article copies available for a fee from The Haworth Document Delivery Service: 1-800-HAWORTH. E-mail address: <docdelivery@haworthpress.com> Website: <http://www.HaworthPress.com>* © *2007 by The Haworth Press, Inc. All rights reserved.]*

KEYWORDS. Prevention, community, engagement, child abuse

INTRODUCTION

The growing body of evidence linking neighborhood characteristics to child well-being has prompted inquiry into identifying the specific pathways that connect these two factors. Neighborhood conditions have been found to significantly influence child maltreatment rates (Garbarino & Sherman, 1980), juvenile delinquency (Brody et al., 2001), early child behavior problems (Linares et al., 2001), and later deviance (Simons et al., 2002). Clearly, neighborhoods, whether defined by statistical units such as census block groups (Coulton, Korbin, & Su, 1999; Simons et al., 2002), or by residents' perceptions (Garbarino, Kostelny, & Dubrow,

1991), influence the developmental trajectory of children. The research on how neighborhoods shape these developmental pathways, however, is less well-developed (Burton & Jarrett, 2000; Leventhal & Brooks-Gunn, 2003). One proposed explanation identifies parenting behavior as a key mechanism linking neighborhood conditions to child development. This explanation suggests that the neighborhood environment shapes the options parents have with respect to their own lives and the lives of their children (Chaskin, 1997). These options, in turn, may influence parenting practices, the home environment (Leventhal & Brooks-Gunn, 2003), and the availability of parenting resources (Jencks & Mayer, 1990)–all of which may produce individual or collective effects on children.

A parent's ability to successfully utilize parenting assistance represents a key resource for meeting the parental needs as well as the needs of their children (see Burton & Jarrett, 2000). Securing answers to questions, accessing tangible assistance in meeting basic needs, and obtaining emotional support for mediating the stress and uncertainty that accompany infant and toddler care can be facilitated or hindered by the proximate availability of local services. Even if such resources are available within one's community, effectively utilizing them may require parents to be proactive in identifying services and overcoming an array of access barriers. At least one study suggests that parents living in communities with low levels of social organization perceive their community as possessing lower quality resources than parents living in more organized communities (Coulton et al., 1999). Such perceptions may discourage parents from seeking support with respect to their parenting concerns.

This study examined the potential role various community attributes might play in influencing a parent's decision to utilize one key resource: voluntary home visitation services. Our analytic sample was drawn from 343 new parents offered services by 1 of 9 Healthy Families America® (HFA) programs that participated in a large applied research effort examining the role of various individual, program and contextual factors on enrollment and retention decisions (Daro, McCurdy, Nelson, Falconnier, & Winje, 2004). Guided by an integrated theory of parent participation (McCurdy & Daro, 2001), this larger effort tested a number of hypotheses related to the decision-making process new parents undergo at various points in the service engagement process. This specific paper reports on those findings related to the role community factors may play in service utilization. Specifically, we test the belief that low levels of social organization in a community will contribute to a parent receiving fewer home visits from a service model designed to support parents and prevent child maltreatment.

Community, Parenting, and Child Maltreatment

The varied effects of parent education efforts across different communities have led programs to broaden their service focus to include improving conditions and service capacity in the communities in which program participants live. Commenting on the positive results from targeted early intervention programs noted by Olds and his colleagues (1998), Felton Earls emphasized this point by speculating on "how much stronger the effects of this early intervention would have been if the program had continued beyond the child's second year of life or *if efforts had been made to engage the wider social settings in which the families lived* [italics added]" (Earls, 1998, p. 1272).

Neighborhood context has long been viewed as an important mediating variable in explaining differential levels of maltreatment among neighborhoods that share a common socioeconomic profile. In a study of neighborhoods in Omaha, Nebraska, Garbarino and Sherman (1980) found that community characteristics significantly explained differential rates of child maltreatment reports. Replicating this methodology with two economically comparable neighborhoods in Washington State, Deccio, Horner, and Wilson (1991) found reported rates of child maltreatment more than two times higher in the community with the higher rate of social disorganization, as evidenced by higher unemployment rates and greater residential mobility.

Community social organization. Coulton and her colleagues at Case Western Reserve University have taken the lead in attempting to specify the connection between urban neighborhood conditions and child maltreatment rates by focusing on the role of community social organization (Coulton, Korbin, Su, & Chow, 1995; Coulton et al., 1999). In their framework, social organization represents the number and connections between and across social networks and neighborhood institutions within a community. These connections are seen as critical for guiding, protecting, and assisting community members, especially children. Low social organization is believed to hinder the establishment of the formal and informal support networks that may be critical in creating a sense of community or trust (Putnam, 1995).

In applying this framework, Coulton et al. (1995) found that neighborhood rates of child maltreatment were significantly linked to macro-level indicators of social organization. The two most significant dimensions identified by this study were neighborhood impoverishment (what we call *distress*), as measured by high rates of poverty, unemployment rates, female-headed households, neighborhood instability, and minority concentration; and what is known as the dependency ratio or a low ratio of caregivers (e.g., adults) to dependent members of the community (e.g., elderly and children). A replication of this study with suburban communities supported the relationship between higher rates of child maltreatment and low social organization, as measured by economic disadvantage (Ernst, 2001).

Though nascent, research suggests that adverse community conditions negatively influence aspects of parental attitudes and behavior. Even after controlling for the effects of maternal education and other indicators of a family's socioeconomic status, studies note a significant relationship between neighborhood impoverishment and more punitive parenting attitudes (Coulton et al., 1999), reduced maternal warmth and harsher parenting practices (Pinderhughes, Foster, Jones, & the Conduct Problems Prevention Research Group, 2001). Further, low levels of social organization have been found to constrain adults and parents from intervening to reduce risky or aversive behavior by others (Garbarino & Kostelny, 1992; Korbin & Coulton, 1997; Sampson, Raudenbush, & Earls, 1997; Wilson, 1987), thereby decreasing the community's role in monitoring and modeling appropriate behavior. Finally, a study by Garbarino and Kostelny reported higher rates of physical abuse by parents living in resource poor, high-risk communities as compared to similar parents in resource adequate, high-risk communities.

Community, Parenting and Service Utilization

The current study seeks to further explicate the mechanisms that connect community, parenting and adverse child outcomes by investigating whether community context influences parental access and use of supportive services. Borrowing from the work of Coulton and her colleagues (1995), we posit that the macro-level indicators of neighborhood social organization found to significantly explain differentials in neighborhood child maltreatment rates also will explain a parent's willingness to utilize parenting support services. Our theoretical model suggests that pervasive and overt negative conditions within a community may deter residents from seeking out or utilizing voluntary services. Such conditions may make residents fearful of exploring service options or may indicate a more general lack of community cohesion or trust (Garbarino & Kostelny, 1992). When the majority of residents are living in poverty, such communities can become increasingly isolated from vibrant commercial centers and high-quality public institutions and resources (Halpern, 1990). In addition, if the number of adults available to care for the more vulnerable or dependent residents in a community is limited, these caretakers may have limited access to other people or resources that can help foster a positive parent-child relationship.

In this study, we test the hypothesis that low levels of community social organization will predict lower parental participation rates in home visiting programs above and beyond the explanatory power of other participant characteristics and services experiences. More specifically, we posit that the parents who live in areas characterized by higher levels of community distress and lower dependency ratios will receive fewer home visits than those parents living in more socially organized neighborhoods.

METHOD

As suggested by our integrated theory and prior work, families will seek out and enroll in voluntary services for myriad reasons that cross several conceptual levels. Further, many of the characteristics that attract families to a given service are not independent of each other. The home visitor's personal skills, although an important factor in determining service quality, will be bounded and influenced by the characteristics of the organization in which she works and by the resources available within her community. Consistent with our theoretical orientation, we have utilized hierarchical linear modeling (HLM) in our past work to examine these types of interdependencies with both a retrospective (Daro, McCurdy, Falconnier, & Stojanovic, 2003) and prospective sample (Daro et al., 2004). Limited sample size and other factors as outlined below, however, precluded the use of HLM techniques in this analysis. As such, we are not able to determine the specific influence of community characteristics within a model that controls for the inevitable contributions of specific provider and program characteristics. However, the methods utilized in this analysis do allow us to determine the added explanatory power of community variables after controlling for a range of participant characteristics and program experiences.

Sample Selection

Study participants were recruited from all new parents who were offered the opportunity to enroll in one of 9 Healthy Families America (HFA) programs across the country between January 2001 and March 2002. The HFA programs were selected, in part, as a convenience sample. All programs were independently evaluated, each evaluator was an active member of an HFA Research Network, and each program had collected data examining questions of model implementation and fidelity. In addition, these programs had been accepting participants for at least 3 years, demonstrating stability of services. The nine programs served families in six states: Arizona, Georgia, Florida, New York, Oregon and Wisconsin.

Each program enrolled consecutive eligible parents until a minimum of 30 families had agreed to the study. Of the 430 families eligible for HFA services, 344 (80%) agreed to participate and provided informed consent, an acceptance rate commonly reported in evaluations of similar programs (Gomby, Culross, & Behrman, 1999). For purposes of this current analysis, our sample was limited to the 307 individuals who had received at least one home visit within 3 months of being offered the intervention. This decision is in keeping with our overall theoretical model that posits that community factors will be exerted on retention rather than enrollment decisions (McCurdy & Daro, 2001). Because this paper examines the relative influence of community characteristics over and above a participant's program experience or attitude toward their home visitor, 49 additional cases were excluded from our analysis due to a lack of information regarding the respondent's address (seven cases) or a lack of sufficient information on the participant's program experience or service provider (42 cases). This resulted in a final potential sample of 258.

As outlined below, our description of a participant's "community" is based on descriptive characteristics provided through the U.S. Census. Although we had initially assumed that each HFA program would draw its participants from a fairly tightly defined geographic area, serving families clustered in a small number of block groups, this did not prove to be the case. The 258 participants in our sample resided in a total of 182 block groups. Of these block groups, 135 or 74% had only one participant. To insure that the variable values across individual subjects were statistically independent, we limited our sample to one participant per block group. For those groups with multiple participants, the participant who enrolled first in the study was retained in the analysis, resulting in a final sample of 182. Although this strategy reduced sample size, a statistical comparison (not shown) of the final sample of 182 and the full sample of all those who received a home visit found no significant differences in demographic characteristics, presenting problems or service experiences.

Procedures

Participants were interviewed within 2 weeks of the HFA enrollment process and 3 months later. For those who remained enrolled at the

3-month point, an additional interview was conducted at 12 months post-enrollment or within 1 month of service termination. Unless otherwise noted, the data used in these analyses came from the measures administered to participants at the initial or 3-month interview. Data on the dependent variable, number of home visits, were drawn from interview data with each participant's home visitor at the time services terminated or 12 months following enrollment.

Measures of Community Social Organization

Our unit of analysis for "community" was a participant's block group, as defined by the U.S. Census. According to the U.S. Census (2003), block groups are contiguous blocks within a census tract that average approximately 1,500 people, though this size ranges from 600 to 3,000 individuals. As noted above, the 258 participants in our sample lived in 182 census block groups. Only one of the programs (the most urban site) averaged more than two service participants per block group (3.5) with all of the other sites averaging between one and two participants per block group. Programs varied in the number of individual block groups they served, ranging from 12 for one inner-city site to 27 for a program targeted to a rural community in the Northwest. Although we recognize that this definition of neighborhood is statistical and may not correspond to a participant's personal definition of their community, this unit of analysis ensured uniformity of definition and reliable access to a wide range of descriptive variables on each participant's immediate residential community.

Community distress. In defining a community's level of social organization, we drew on the methodology adopted by the Working Group on Communities, Neighborhoods, Family Process and Individual Development (Brooks-Gunn, Duncan, & Aber, 1997). As noted earlier, this research identified a number of macro-level indicators that correlate with community child maltreatment rates. Using the 2000 U.S. Census data (2003), we conducted a factor analysis on a wide range of variables commonly used to denote social or economic stress to determine the best fit between our conceptual interests and internal consistency. After considering a range of options, we identified a set of variables that formed a strong construct which we labeled "community distress" ($\alpha = .87$). The specific variables included in this scale are: the percent of residents with less than a high school education; the percent of unemployed males 16 or older; the percent of non-white residents; the percent of rental households; the percent of households with incomes under $20,000; the percent of female-headed households; and the percent of households receiving SSI and/or public assistance. Mean scores on this scale across the 182 block groups ranged from 11 to over 60 (out of a possible score of 100), with higher scores denoting greater distress.

Dependency ratio. Drawing on the work of Coulton, Korbin and their colleagues (1995), we also computed the dependency ratio for each census block group (e.g., the number of individuals under age 18 or over age 65 divided by the number of individuals between ages 19 and 64). This measure served as a proxy of the pool of individuals potentially able to provide support to children, the elderly and their families. Higher scores denote a larger proportion of children and elderly in need of care relative to the number of potential caretakers. The mean scores across all of the census block groups in this sample ranged from slightly greater than 1 to less than .10.

Participant-Level Independent Variables

Demographic characteristics. Descriptive characteristics were drawn from the initial participant interviews and included race/ethnicity and a count of the number of demographic or socioeconomic factors that may place a new mother at an elevated risk for child abuse. The participant's score on this risk index included the number of affirmative responses to each of the following conditions: not married; unemployed and not in school; 20 years of age or younger; and not yet completed high school or received a GED. This process of summarizing risk conditions has been used in the national evaluation of the early Head Start Program (Love et al., 2001). Values ranged from 0 (the participant had none of the characteristics) to 4 (the participant had all of the characteristics).

Presenting concerns and resources. Three variables were used to summarize the concerns facing participants and their level of potential support from their informal network. First, the *infant risk* measure notes the number of specific conditions the infant experienced at the time of birth. The value for this measure ranged from 0 to 4 and represents the number of affirmative responses the mother provided at the 3-month interview (or the first post-birth interview) to the existence of the following conditions: premature birth, baby not held after birth, low birth weight, use of special nursery. In our analysis, this variable was recoded to indicate if the participant reported no risk factors for their baby (0) or at least one risk factor (1). Second, the *total concern measure* is the total number of positive responses (0-12) a participant provided during the 3-month interview to whether the following issues were of concern to them: feeding her baby, getting health care for the baby, finding a job, paying her bills, finding better housing, finding child care, relationship with her partner or spouse, relationship with parents, relationship with her child, going to school, or making friends in the community.

With respect to the availability of support from family members and friends, participants were asked a series of questions at the initial interview regarding the availability of support from three sources (e.g., father of the baby or current partner, family members or relatives, friends or neighborhoods). For each source, the participant indicated if they expected assistance in each of five specific areas: information on child rearing, getting things for the baby, finding a doctor for the baby, getting the baby to the doctor, or getting connected to other parents. Values on the *availability of informal support* measure were the number of positive responses to these questions and ranged from 0 (no support from any sources) to 17 (a variety of supports from a variety of sources).

Participant view of program. Four individual variables were identified to capture the participant's response to or perception of home visitation services at the time of the 3-month interview. First, participants were asked to rate how individuals in their informal network (e.g., partner, father of the baby, relatives or friends) felt about their involvement in the program on a 5-point Likert scale, with 1 indicating *very much against* enrollment and 5 indicating *very much for* enrollment. Values for the *personal network supports program* variable were the average level of support for enrollment reported across various members of a participant's network.

Second, participants were asked if they perceived that the program had changed their attitudes or behaviors in four specific areas (e.g., what they know about being a parent, the information available to them on what to expect from their child, the way they act as a parent, and other ways on a personal or parenting level). Values for the *program changed participant* variable were the mean response to all four areas and ranged from 0 (program had no impact on any of the four areas) to 1 (program had an impact on all four areas).

Third, participants were asked to respond to a series of descriptive statements regarding their relationship with their home visitor on a 5-point scale where 1 indicated they *strongly disagreed* with the statement and 5 indicated that they *strongly agreed* with the statement. Eight of these items referred to the extent to which a participant felt the home visitor respected her family's beliefs and culture and encouraged her to utilize her family network and other sources of community support in addressing her parenting needs (e.g., the FSW accepts my family as important people who help me to parent, the FSW encourages us to value our progress, etc.). These items, which we labeled *FSW support scale*, produced a scale with strong internal consistency (α = .81).

Finally, the *Helping Relationship Inventory* is a standardized assessment of the quality of the participant-provider relationship (Poulin & Young, 1997; Young & Poulin, 1998). The participant version includes 10 items that address the structural component of the service interaction (e.g., the process for identifying the family's service goals, the clarity of the program's objectives, the methods for assessing progress, etc.) and 10 items addressing the interpersonal component of service delivery (e.g., the extent to which the relationship was mutually satisfying, the emotional connection between participant and provider, the impact of the intervention on attitudes and feelings, etc.). The higher the absolute score, the more positive the respondent's view of the relationship. Scoring for this 20-item measure is the mean response participants provided to each question on a 5-point Likert scale, where 1 indicated the statement was *not at all* reflective of the participants' experiences and 5 indicated the statement was *a great deal* reflective of their experiences. The internal consistency of this measure for the study population was very high (α = .81).

Dependent Variable

Our broader examination of retention issues has utilized two measures of engagement, both of which were provided by the participant's home visitor: the number of visits a participant received and the length of time the participant received services. As our results have been similar across these two outcomes, this paper presents the results of the analyses utilizing number of visits. On average, participants in this sample received 17.18 visits (SD = 13.08), ranging from 1 to 60, during the first year of program participation.

Analysis

Standard OLS multiple regression techniques were used to examine the unique contribution of community characteristics in explaining a new parent's use of voluntary home visitation programs. Specifically, all of the participant level factors were entered in four blocks–demographic characteristics, presenting problems and strengths, program experiences, and community characteristics. We apply a conservative test of community characteristics by entering the community variables in the last block to asses the portion of additional variance explained by community attributes after accounting for all other factors in the model.

RESULTS

Participant Characteristics

Table 1 summarizes the characteristics of the 182 participants in our sample by program. Overall, approximately one-third of the study participants were African American, one-third White and 20% Hispanic. The remainder of the sample, 6%, included several Native American participants from Program I and participants indicating a mixed ethnic/racial identity from Program B. At the individual program level, far less diversity was observed in the ethnic identity of the participant population, with over 50% of the participants from eight of the nine sites coming from a single ethnic group.

In terms of presenting risk factors, these participants carried, on average, two of the four demographic markers generally associated with an elevated risk for parental stress (e.g., single parent status, less than a high school education, young maternal age, and unemployed but not in school). Overall, one third of these participants were teen parents. Most participants were involved with a partner (51%) or married (an additional 14%) and over 80% were not employed or in school at the time HFA services were offered. In terms of educational attainment, 55% of the sample had not yet received a high school diploma or GED, perhaps reflecting the high proportion of teen participants.

At the time of enrollment in the study, the average participant identified between three and four parenting concerns regarding such issues as basic infant care, employment or economic security, securing adequate health care or housing, and relationships with their partner or child. Looking across the nine programs, the average number of concerns ranged from a high of 5.6 at Program F to a low of 1.8 at Program A, underscoring the variability in the needs of families served by the HFA model. Similarly, although about one-third of all participants identified at least one initial concern regarding their infant's health, this proportion ranged from 57% at Program E to 20% at Program B. In terms of protective factors, the average participant in this sample was able to identify a moderate number of informal support resources among their network of family members and friends, scoring on average 7.6 on this 17-point scale. Again, we observed

TABLE 1. Participant Characteristics by Program

Program	Sample	Race				Risks and Protective Factors				Program Experiences				
		% AA	% White	% Hispanic	% Other	Mean SES Risk (SD)	% Infant Risk	Mean Total Concerns (SD)	Mean Informal Support (SD)	Mean Network Support for HFA (SD)	% Reporting Change By HFA	Mean FSW Support/ Network (SD)	Mean HRI score (SD)	Mean # Home Visits
A	11	18	18	64	0	2.18 (0.75)	27	1.82 (1.77)	6.55 (3.80)	3.92 (0.32)	41	3.85 (0.27)	3.50 (0.69)	10.09 (7.19)
B	15	40	27	13	20	1.67 (0.72)	20	2.33 (2.16)	7.13 (3.04)	4.10 (0.60)	63	4.00 (0.43)	3.71 (0.53)	11.00 (7.04)
C	25	84	12	4	0	1.84 (0.55)	28	3.52 (2.10)	8.64 (3.56)	4.12 (0.49)	32	3.96 (0.29)	3.31 (0.83)	16.76 (11.69)
D	22	77	14	9	0	2.14 (0.71)	45	3.91 (2.50)	10.86 (3.04)	3.99 (0.55)	56	4.22 (0.63)	3.51 (1.14)	7.86 (9.59)
E	19	74	5	16	5	2.00 (0.75)	57	3.16 (2.69)	9.58 (3.38)	4.18 (0.55)	56	4.12 (0.56)	3.86 (0.73)	29.37 (10.45)
F	12	0	0	100	0	2.08 (0.29)	33	5.58 (3.31)	6.33 (3.06)	4.02 (0.49)	71	4.14 (0.28)	3.62 (0.72)	36.92 (10.55)
G	27	7	63	22	7	1.78 (0.70)	25	3.93 (2.78)	5.00 (2.76)	4.06 (0.61)	50	4.09 (0.45)	3.51 (0.65)	15.11 (10.62)
H	26	4	81	15	0	2.23 (0.91)	42	3.50 (2.60)	7.69 (2.87)	4.05 (0.58)	63	4.04 (0.49)	3.38 (0.72)	11.73 (11.33)
I	25	16	56	8	20	1.96 (0.73)	36	3.72 (1.77)	6.52 (3.66)	3.95 (0.54)	47	4.18 (0.43)	3.63 (0.76)	21.80 (11.71)
Full sample	182	37	36	21	6	1.97 (0.72)	36	3.55 (2.52)	7.64 (3.63)	4.05 (0.54)	52	4.08 (0.49)	3.54 (0.78)	17.18 (13.09)

variation on this indicator across the nine programs, with average informal support levels ranging from a score of 5 to almost 10.

The participants' informal support networks were generally supportive of HFA service, As noted in Table 1, average scores on this scale across the programs ranged between 3.9 and 4.2 on a 5-point scale, with a score of 5 indicating strong support. About half of the sample indicated that their involvement in HFA services changed their parenting attitudes or behaviors, with this proportion varying from a high of 71% in Program F to a low of 32% in Program C. This self-assessment of progress was significantly and moderately correlated with the number of visits a participant received ($r = .22$, $p = .004$). The participants served by each site received, on average, between eight to 37 home visits, again underscoring the variability in HFA service levels across programs.

On the FSW support scale, participants reported positive relationships with their home visitor and indicated that their family support workers demonstrated a respect for their belief system and encouraged them to use informal supports and community resources in addressing their personal and parenting concerns. Scores on the HRI scale indicated moderate satisfaction with the structure of the home visits and a belief that the participant was active in shaping her service options and respected by the visitor. Although some variation on both measures existed across the nine programs, average scores for all of the sites were at the more favorable end of the response continuum on both measures.

Community Characteristics

Table 2 summarizes the variation in the community characteristics represented across the nine HFA program sites. Reflective of HFA's commitment to providing a wide range of parents access to support services, the target areas served by this pool of programs represent a diverse set of communities. Although analysis of variance detected significantly greater between-programs than within-program variance, many of the participants resided in contiguous block groups that often differed in terms of socioeconomic profile and neighborhood conditions. Census data across all block groups indicated that approximately 20% of the residents were judged to be living in poverty, a proportion that ranged from a high of 36% to a low of 9%. One-third of all of the households with children in these communities were headed by single mothers, a proportion that varied from over half in two of the sites to less than one-quarter in four of the sites. The proportion of children living within two parent/adult households ranged from less than half to over three-quarters. Almost one-third of the residents in these

TABLE 2. Community Characteristics by Program

Program	# of Block Groups	Mean Population (SD)	Mean % Population Under 5 (SD)	Mean % Population Identified as living in poverty (SD)	Mean % households w/ children female headed (SD)	Mean % households w/ children married couples (SD)	Mean % ≥25 lacking HS/GED (SD)	Mean % ≥25 BA, MA or Ph.D. (SD)	Mean Distress Score (SD)	Mean Dependency Score (SD)
					Household Characteristics		Education			
A	11	2,241 (903)	9 (1.76)	21 (11.88)	23 (8.16)	68 (9.83)	36 (16.12)	10 (9.68)	37.6 (10.1)	.81 (0.12)
B	15	1,633 (1,085)	7 (1.68)	19 (10.44)	32 (9.74)	57 (10.23)	22 (10.88)	15 (5.74)	37.4 (9.05)	.65 (0.14)
C	25	1,213 (925)	7 (1.98)	26 (9.03)	46 (12.81)	45 (12.38)	35 (11.42)	8 (5.90)	47.0 (7.78)	.73 (0.15)
D	22	2,547 (1,216)	8 (1.22)	11 (7.50)	35 (13.45)	57 (13.33)	19 (12.91)	25 (14.23)	35.4 (9.43)	.53 (0.10)
E	19	1,322 (1,025)	8 (1.66)	23 (15.72)	34 (14.11)	59 (14.94)	29 (14.90)	12 (10.47)	40.0 (11.74)	.65 (0.11)
F	12	2,160 (719)	7 (1.20)	36 (6.68)	48 (4.93)	42 (4.30)	56 (7.86)	7 (3.24)	61.0 (3.31)	.55 (0.08)
G	27	2,170 (1,381)	7 (2.18)	9 (5.15)	17 (6.28)	76 (8.68)	15 (9.57)	25 (16.45)	29.2 (12.21)	.61 (0.09)
H	26	1,703 (808)	6 (1.89)	19 (14.21)	21 (8.30)	71 (10.93)	17 (9.21)	19 (14.12)	30.2 (6.67)	.57 (0.17)
I	25	1,574 (1,512)	7 (1.84)	14 (7.94)	24 (7.54)	66 (10.75)	21 (9.76)	15 (8.22)	34.1 (6.18)	.57 (0.13)
Full Sample	182	1,806 (1,190)	7 (1.86)	19 (12.42)	30 (14.15)	61 (15.45)	25 (15.69)	16 (12.78)	37.5 (12.09)	.62 (0.15)

195

block groups lacked a high school diploma or equivalent level of education and roughly 16% of those over 25 had a college degree, statistics that also varied considerably across the nine program sites.

Capturing this type of variance, average scores on our overall measure of community distress ranged from a high of 61 to a low of 29 and the proportion of potential caregivers to those in need of care ranged from .53 to .81.

Regression Findings

Table 3 presents the multiple regression results. The final model indicates that all variables, taken together, explained 21% ($p < .001$) of the total variance in the number of home visits provided this HFA participant sample. In the first block, 1% of the variance in home visits was captured by the participants' demographic characteristics; the addition of initial risk and protective factors in the second block explains an additional 4% of the variance ($p < .01$). In the third block, entering program experiences increases the explained variance by 8% ($p < .001$). As expected, the inclusion of community factors in the fourth block adds a further 8% ($p < .001$) to the explained variance.

In the final model, non-community factors across a variety of areas emerged as significant predictors of home visits. Race was the only demographic variable to achieve a significant ($p < .05$) effect. African American participants received fewer home visits than non-African American participants, a relationship that remained constant even when we independently compared the performance of African American participants to the two other major ethnic groups (e.g., Hispanics and Whites) represented in the sample.

Two presenting concerns, infant risk and total concerns, significantly influenced the receipt of visits. Participants giving birth to infants presenting at least one indicator of risk (e.g., low birth weight, placed in a special nursery following birth, etc.) received a greater number of home visits than participants giving birth to infants with no presenting risk factors. Participants who reported a greater number of parenting and personal concerns at three months following enrollment received a greater number of home visits than participants with fewer concerns. In addition, there was a trend ($p < .07$) for participants with larger informal support networks to receive fewer home visits than those with smaller networks.

Of the program experiences posited to impact participation, only the relationship with the home visitor achieved significance ($p < .01$). Participants assessing the relationship as more positive received more

TABLE 3. Multiple Regression Analysis Predicting Number of Home Visits

Variable	Step 1			Step 2			Step 3			Step 4		
	B	SE	β	B	SE	β	B	SE	β	B	SE	β
(Constant)	18.9	3.0		15.5	3.8		-3.6	9.9		-15.4	11.2	
Participant Characteristics												
SES Risk Index	-0.2	1.3	-.01	-0.1	1.3	-.01	0.2	1.3	.01	0.4	1.2	.02
African American	-3.5	2.0	-.13[a]	-2.5	2.1	-.09	-2.3	2.0	-.08	-4.3	2.0	-.16*
Presenting Concerns												
Infant Risk				3.8	2.0	.14[a]	4.6	1.9	.17*	4.7	1.9	.17**
Total Concerns				1.1	0.4	.20**	1.1	0.4	.21**	0.8	.36	.16*
Available Informal support				-0.3	0.3	-.08	-0.5	0.3	-.13[a]	-0.5	.26	-.13[a]
Program Experiences												
Support for HFA among participant's network							2.5	1.8	.10	2.8	1.7	.12[a]
Program changed participant							1.6	3.5	.04	0.5	3.3	.01
FSW encourages use of informal supports							-2.1	2.4	-.08	-1.1	2.3	-.04
HRI average score							4.9	1.7	.29**	4.0	1.6	.24**
Community Factors												
Dependency ratio										-2.0	6.5	-.02
Community distress										0.3	0.8	.31***
F change	1.55			2.98**			4.02***			5.33***		
df	181			181			181			181		
Adjusted R^2	.01			.05			.13			.21		

[a] $p < .10$, * $p < .05$, ** $p < .01$, *** $p < .001$

197

visits than those with less positive relationships. A trend did emerge such that participants received more visits if their informal network support system was perceived as supportive of HFA services ($p < .11$).

In terms of our community variables, only the measure of community distress had a significant impact on the number of home visits participants received. Contrary to our initial assumption, residents in the communities with the greatest level of distress received more, not fewer, home visits. Also, our hypothesis that lower dependency ratios would correspond to fewer visits was not supported. Dependency ratios did not significantly impact receipt of visits.

DISCUSSION

Major Findings

Despite its universal outreach, a certain efficiency appears to exist among HFA programs in how home visiting services are allocated, with the greatest number of home visits being provided to new parents with the highest-risk infants, the fewest social supports, and who live in the most distressed communities. Our analysis suggests that key factors in achieving this efficiency may be both the targeting of high-risk communities as well as the nature of the provider-participant relationship. Specifically, HFA's universal outreach to new parents living in neighborhoods with moderate to high levels of distress may bring a welcomed service opportunity to families who struggle with finding the few available resources that may exist in their local community. By introducing the option of on-going assistance, the HFA approach does not require new parents to self-identify as being in need of support. This type of normalization of the helping process has been advocated by others as an essential component for enhancing the success of prevention and early intervention efforts (Melton & Berry, 1994).

Successfully enrolling residents living in high-risk communities in HFA programs, however, might hinge on the home visitor's ability to engage families in the case planning process and the family's ability to respond to these types of incentives. In our model, those participants who rated their relationship with their worker as involving more active participation in the case planning process received more home visits. This strategy of actively engaging a participant in defining her needs and determining her case plan may increase the likelihood she will keep scheduled appointments. Participants who have a more passive relationship with their home visitor may remain on a program's caseload, but may not be highly motivated to help insure that an actual home visit occurs.

Study Limitations

As with all research, this analysis is limited to a specific set of HFA programs, with a specific set of participants, over a specific period of time. Given the evolving nature of community-based programs like HFA, one that is guided by a theoretical model incorporating ongoing program improvement based on emerging data, many of the strategies or experiences documented by the participants in this study may not be fully representative of current HFA practice. A second limitation concerns our definition of community. Like others, we utilized census data to define neighborhood; however, it is likely that a U.S. census tract may not reflect the boundaries individual participants would place on what they consider to be their "neighborhood." Further, the use of census data limited our neighborhood assessments to general descriptive data which, while often associated with key indicators of community distress and disorganization, cannot capture how individual participants view the quality of their neighborhood. Relying on these types of broad, aggregate characteristics may not provide the kind and quality of information needed to address the more complex question as to how individual families draw on community resources or feel limited by community characteristics in meeting their parenting obligations.

This analysis was not able to take into account the unique contributions of key provider and program characteristics we have identified in our earlier work as contributing to participant enrollment and retention decisions. Although hierarchical linear modeling (HLM) has been used by ourselves and others to address the methodological challenge of working with nested data, we are not convinced that the application of this method produces stable and robust findings with relatively small samples. Using HLM techniques to detect the relative influence of specific variables at participant, provider, program and community levels may require samples of sufficient size across all levels of a given analytic model in order to provide the degree of variation necessary to reliably identify the most salient explanatory factors after controlling for the contributions of each previous level.

Implications for Practice

A common assumption in assessing community-based services is that such services are offered to residents who share a similar neighborhood context and geographic location and are, therefore, more "place-based" than large public social service or health providers. Indeed, the majority of HFA programs around the country explicitly target their services to a specific census tract or neighborhood. Our data suggest, however, that this assumption may mask wide variation in the neighborhood realities for families served by a single program. Once HFA programs move out of large urban areas, it is not uncommon for them to serve a set of communities that often differ from each other in terms of socioeconomic status and human resources. Rather than viewing a program as serving a specific community, HFA program managers and providers need to plan for serving several communities within their target area. To better engage this range of families, HFA programs need to acquire knowledge of the varying neighborhood conditions and resources, and an ability to adapt staffing patterns and service delivery procedures to the unique community where the participant resides.

The distress level in a local community may have both positive and negative impacts on the willingness of families to seek out and engage in voluntary services as well as the ability of organizations to provide family support services. In this study, parents in highly distressed communities were more likely to receive visits. Other studies, however, note that such communities can present significant challenges to program managers in securing a stable work force and in meeting the service needs of parents (Love et al., 2002). Clearly, our results indicate that programs can successfully target highly distressed communities despite the many challenges presented by such communities.

Our earlier work in examining retention rates among HFA participants led us to suggest that the agencies most successful in retaining families and delivering the greatest number of home visits were embedded in community support agencies and tended to employ a high proportion of experienced workers who placed high value on involving families in the service planning process (Daro et al., 2003). The findings in this study further accentuate the importance of the provider-parent relationship noted by others (Korfmacher, 1998). Programs hoping to engage similar participants should offer specific training aimed at ways for visitors to *guide* service planning and delivery, and to avoid strategies that tend to prescribe service delivery.

Implications for Research

The evidence regarding how community context influences adult behaviors is starting to accumulate. Some evidence suggests that neighborhood disadvantage correlates with negative adult behaviors, such as increased likelihood of partner violence (Cunradi, Caetano, Clark, & Schafer, 2000), and increased rate of subsequent pregnancies among welfare recipients (Gold et al., 2005). However, one study reports that, for African-American families, living in disadvantaged communities results in higher marital quality than living in more advantaged communities (Cutrona et al., 2003). Additional research which draws on observational data regarding neighborhood quality and personal interactions is needed to better specify the way community influences parenting norms as well as the capacity of individuals to seek out and utilize family support services.

Our findings that ethnicity influenced participation rates highlight another area in need of further research. In the current study, African-American participants received fewer visits than European Americans or Latinas. While these findings are somewhat in line with research on center-based, therapeutic interventions (Wierzbicki & Pekarik, 1993), they contrast with more recent studies of home visiting programs that found similar or higher rates of participation by African Americans as compared to whites (McCurdy, Gannon, & Daro, 2003; Navaie-Waliser et al., 2000). Indeed, engagement patterns among this same sample indicated that African-American and Hispanic participants were more likely to enroll in home visiting services than white participants (McCurdy et al., in press). As communities in the United States are becoming increasingly segregated by income and race (Iceland, 2003), future analyses of community effects will need to disentangle the relationship among community, ethnicity, and income.

CONCLUSIONS

Participants do seek out, enroll and remain in voluntary services in part because of their own characteristics and preferences. However, these choices also are influenced by their program experiences and relationships with their home visitor. In addition, community context does matter but not in the direction we had assumed. Once enrolled, new parents living in the most distressed communities are far more likely to receive a greater number of visits than those in less distressed areas. Certain features of the HFA service model may facilitate its implementation within high-risk communities and contribute to its ability to achieve strong service levels in areas that can be inhospitable to social service interventions. These features include the delivery of services within a participant's home, the ability to assess and respond to a broad range of parenting and personal concerns, and the use of home visitors who encourage participants to draw on their informal support services and to be active participants in the service planning process.

REFERENCES

Brody, G., Ge, X., Conger, R., Gibbons, F., McBride, V., Cerrard, M. et al. (2001). The influence of neighborhood disadvantage, collective socialization, and parenting on African-American children's affiliation with deviant peers. *Child Development, 72,* 1231-1246.

Brooks-Gunn, J., Duncan, G., & Aber, J. L. (1997). *Neighborhood poverty. Volume II: Policy implications in studying neighborhoods.* New York: Russell Sage Foundation.

Burton, L. M., & Jarrett, R. L. (2000). In the mix, yet on the margins: The place of families in urban neighborhood and child development research. *Journal of Marriage and the Family, 62,* 1114-1135.

Chaskin, R. (1997). Perspectives on neighborhood and community: A review of the literature. *Social Service Review, 71,* 521-547.

Coulton, C. J., Korbin, J. E., & Su, M. (1999). Neighborhoods and child maltreatment: A multi-level study. *Child Abuse and Neglect, 23,* 1019-1040.

Coulton, C. J., Korbin, J. E., Su, M., & Chow, J. (1995). Community level factors and child maltreatment rates. *Child Development, 66,* 1262-1276.

Cunradi, C., Caetano, R., Clark, C., & Schafer, J. (2000). Neighborhood poverty as a predictor of intimate partner violence among white, black and Hispanic couples in the United States: A multilevel analysis. *Annals of Epidemiology, 10,* 297-308.

Cutrona, C., Russell, D., Abraham, W. T., Kardner, K., Melby, J., Bryant, C. et al. (2003). Neighborhood context and financial strain as predictors of marital interaction and marital quality in African American couples. *Personal Relationships, 10,* 389-409.

Daro, D., McCurdy, K., Falconnier, L., & Stojanovic, D. (2003). Sustaining new parents in home visitation services: Key participant and program factors. *Child Abuse and Neglect, 27,* 1101-1125.

Daro, D., McCurdy, K., Nelson, C., Falconnier, L., & Winje, C. (2004). *Engagement and retention in voluntary new parent support programs.* Final report. Submitted to the W. T. Grant Foundation, New York.

Deccio, G., Horner, B., & Wilson, D. (1991). *High-risk neighborhoods and high-risk families: Replication research related to the human ecology of child maltreatment.* Unpublished manuscript, Eastern Washington University, Cheney, WA.

Earls, F. (1998). Positive effects of prenatal and early childhood interventions. *Journal of the American Medical Association, 280,* 1271-1273.

Ernst, J. S. (2001). Community-level factors and child maltreatment in a suburban community. *Social Work Research, 25,* 133-142.

Garbarino, J., & Kostelny, K. (1992). Child maltreatment as a community problem. *Child Abuse and Neglect, 16,* 455-464.

Garbarino, J., Kostelny, K., & Dubrow, N. (1991). What children can tell us about living in danger. *American Psychologist, 46,* 376-383.

Garbarino, J., & Sherman, D. (1980). High-risk neighborhoods and high-risk families: The human ecology of child maltreatment. *Child Development, 51*, 188-198.

Gold, R., Connell, F., Heagerty, P., Bezruchka, S., Davis, R., & Cawthon, M. L. (2004). Income inequality and pregnancy spacing. *Social Science & Medicine, 59*, 1117-1126.

Gomby, D., Culross, P., & Behrman, R. (1999). Home visiting: Recent program evaluations–analysis and recommendations. *The Future of Children, 9*, 4-26.

Halpern, R. (1990). Poverty and early childhood parenting: Toward a framework for intervention. *American Journal of Orthopsychiatry, 60*, 6-18.

Iceland, J. (2003). *Poverty in America: A handbook*. Berkeley, CA: The University of California Press.

Jencks, C., & Mayer, S. (1990). The social consequences of growing up in a poor neighborhood. In L. Lynn, Jr., & M. McGeary (Eds.), *Inner-city poverty in America* (pp. 111-186). Washington, DC: National Academy Press.

Korbin, J., & Coulton, C. (1997). Understanding the neighborhood context for children and families: Combining epidemiological and ethnographic approaches. In J. Brooks-Gunn, G. Duncan, & J. L. Aber (Eds.), *Neighborhood poverty. Volume II: Policy implications in studying neighborhoods* (pp. 65-79). New York: Russell Sage Foundation.

Korfmacher, J. (1998, February/March). Examining the service provider in early intervention. *Zero to Three*, 17-22.

Leventhal, T., & Brooks-Gunn, J. (2003). Children and youth in neighborhood contexts. *Current Directions in Psychological Science, 12*, 27-31.

Linares, L. O., Heeren, R., Bronfman, E., Zuckerman, B., Augustyn, M., & Tronick, E. (2001). A mediational model for the impact of exposure to community violence on early child behavior problems. *Child Development, 72*, 639-652.

Love, J., Kisker, E., Ross, C., Schochet, P., Brooks-Gunn, J., Paulsell, D. et al. (2002). *Making a difference in the lives of infants and toddlers and their families: The impact of early Head Start*. Report prepared for the U.S. Department of Health and Human Services, Administration of Children and Families.

McCurdy, K., & Daro, D. (2001). Parent involvement in family support programs: An integrated theory. *Family Relations, 50*, 113-121.

McCurdy, K., Daro, D., Anisfeld, E., Katzev, A., Keim, A., LeCroy, C. et al. (in press). Understanding maternal intentions to engage in home visiting programs. *Children and Youth Services Review*.

McCurdy, K., Gannon, R., & Daro, D. (2003). Participation in home-based, family support programs: Ethnic variations. *Family Relations, 52*, 3-11.

Melton, G., & Berry, F. (Eds.) (1994). *Protecting children from abuse and neglect: Foundations for a new national strategy*. New York: Guilford Press.

Navaie-Waliser, M., Martin, S. L., Campbell, M. K., Tessaro, I., Kotelchuck, M., & Cross, A. W. (2000). Factors predicting completion of a home visitation program by high-risk pregnant women: The North Carolina maternal outreach worker program. *American Journal of Public Health, 90*, 121-124.

Olds, D., Henderson, C., Cole, R., Eckenrode, J., Kitzman, H., Luckey, D. et al. (1998). Long-term effects of nurse home visitation on children's criminal and antisocial behavior. *Journal of the American Medical Association, 280*, 1238-1244.

Pinderhughes, E. E., Nix, R., Foster, E. M., & Jones, D. (2001). Parenting in context: Impact of neighborhood poverty, residential stability, public services, social networks, and danger on parental behaviors. *Journal of Marriage and Family, 63,* 941-953.

Poulin, J., & Young, T. (1997). Development of a helping relationship inventory for social work practice. *Research on Social Work Practice, 7,* 463-489.

Putnam, R. (1995). Bowling alone: America's declining social capital. *Journal of Democracy, 6,* 65-78.

Sampson, R., Raudenbush, S., & Earls, F. (1997). Neighborhoods and violent crime: A multilevel study of collective efficacy. *Science, 277,* 918-924.

Simons, R. L., Lin, K. H., Gordon, L. C., Brody, G. H., Murry, V., & Conger, R. D. (2002). Community differences in the association between parenting practice and child conduct problems. *Journal of Marriage and Family, 64,* 331-345.

U.S. Census Bureau (2003). *Census 2000 summary file 3* [Computer software]. Washington, DC.

Wierzbicki, M., & Pekarik, G. (1993). A meta-analysis of psychotherapy dropout. *Professional Psychology: Research and Practice, 24,* 190-195.

Wilson, J. (1987). *The truly disadvantaged: The inner city, the underclass, and public policy.* Chicago: University of Chicago Press.

Young, T., & Poulin, J. (1998). The Helping Relationship Inventory: A clinical appraisal. *Families in Society: The Journal of Contemporary Human Services, 79,* 123-133.

doi:10.1300/J005v34n01_09

Potential Lessons from Public Health
and Health Promotion
for the Prevention of Child Abuse

Joanne B. Martin

Indiana University

Lawrence W. Green

University of California at San Francisco

Andrea Carlson Gielen

Johns Hopkins University

SUMMARY. Two successful public health efforts of the last third of the twentieth century–tobacco control and automobile injury control–are reviewed for relevance to the problem of child abuse. Potential lessons for child abuse prevention are identified and the following approaches are suggested: Investigate varied logic models or conceptual frameworks to identify new opportunities for effective intervention. Use a multi-disciplinary, multi-sector approach. Normalize desired behaviors and denormalize undesirable behaviors. Balance efficacy, feasibility, and

Address correspondence to: Joanne B. Martin, School of Nursing, Indiana University, 1111 Middle Drive, NU 238, Indianapolis, IN 46202-5107 (E-mail: jbmartin@iupui. edu).

[Haworth co-indexing entry note]: "Potential Lessons from Public Health and Health Promotion for the Prevention of Child Abuse." Martin, Joanne B., Lawrence W. Green, and Andrea Carlson Gielen. Co-published simultaneously in *Journal of Prevention & Intervention in the Community* (The Haworth Press, Inc.) Vol. 34. No.1/2, 2007, pp. 205-222; and: *The Healthy Families America® Initiative: Integrating Research, Theory and Practice* (ed: Joseph Galano) The Haworth Press, 2007, pp. 205-222. Single or multiple copies of this article are available for a fee from The Haworth Document Delivery Service [1-800-HAWORTH, 9:00 a.m. - 5:00 p.m. (EST). E-mail address: docdelivery@haworthpress.com].

cultural appropriateness. Develop strategies for effective policy advocacy based upon who benefits and who shoulders most of the burden.
doi:10.1300/J005v34n01_10 *[Article copies available for a fee from The Haworth
Document Delivery Service: 1-800-HAWORTH. E-mail address: <docdelivery@
haworthpress.com> Website: <http://www.HaworthPress.com> © 2007 by The
Haworth Press, Inc. All rights reserved.]*

KEYWORDS. Child abuse, tobacco control, automobile injury control,
public health campaigns, health promotion

INTRODUCTION

In the second half of the 20th century, the science of epidemiology, and
public health strategies of public awareness and action for community
mobilization, consumer protection, environmental engineering, regulation and social policy, developed for infectious disease control, were
adapted to chronic disease control and injury control. Two of the great
successes of the last third of the 20th century in North America–control of
the tobacco epidemic and reduction in auto crashes–each called into
much greater play the role of social and behavioral sciences. These two
were declared by Centers for Disease Control (CDC) to be among the 10
greatest public health achievements of the 20th century (CDC, 1999a).
This review of the tobacco control and auto safety successes will examine
those aspects that could hold particular relevance for improved child
abuse prevention.

THE CASE FOR DRAWING GENERALIZATIONS ACROSS TYPES OF PROGRAMS

Most of the guidance for professional and organizational practices in
planning and implementing programs tends to come from demonstration
or model projects, or better, a rigorous evaluation of them and, at best, the
synthesis of evaluations or randomized trial studies of similar interventions
across multiple sites. Demonstration projects without rigorous evaluation are notoriously susceptible to biases in the conduct and reporting of
results, to the enthusiasm or resources at the disposal of the demonstration
site, and to the difficulties of replicating demonstrations in less favorable
settings. Rigorous evaluations help control for most of the biases, but the
unrepresentative nature of the demonstration site, its resources and its
proponents and staff still make replication difficult, if not impractical.
Evaluations and randomized trials across multiple sites may allay the

problem of a single demonstration site, but still leave many practitioners feeling that research attention and auspices for the demonstration programs render them unrealistic for their local situations (Green, 2001). With these caveats and reservations, some practitioners are more willing to take their guidance and inspiration from obvious successes in other fields than from equivocal or dubious research evidence accumulating gradually in their own field (Lancaster, 1992).

Recognizing that lessons do not flow only in one direction, we ask, however, what lessons from tobacco control and injury prevention might be applied to the field of child abuse prevention? At least four features of the experience in tobacco control and automobile injury control make these two fields of behavioral and environmental interventions similar enough to child abuse prevention to warrant our supposition that success in one might hold lessons for the other.

One, all three involve complex behavioral patterns that typically occur outside the purview of health professionals and yield low rates of success with clinical or individual-level intervention, relative to what clinicians are accustomed to expecting. Two, clinicians lack incentives to change these behaviors. Financial compensation is not commensurate with the time and effort required for any effect. Moreover, clinicians fear they will lose their patient or client if they seem to be nagging and moralizing about the patient's or client's smoking, driving or parenting behavior. Three, all three behaviors can be measured and correlated with other factors surrounding or antecedent to the behavior. Thus it is possible to construct a prevention science that identifies specific points of intervention to curtail the behavior or minimize the adverse impact on health. Four, all three have built upon strong public sentiment and support for protecting children, despite the reluctance of policymakers to intrude on adult behaviors associated with smoking, driving, and parenting.

True, smoking is addictive and driving a vehicle occurs outside the home. Nonetheless, changing deeply rooted behaviors such as parenting is a difficult challenge and most driving does not occur under the watchful eye of law enforcement. The goal is to have people practice healthful behaviors when no one is watching.

THE TOBACCO CONTROL EXPERIENCE

For a long time, health-care professionals and teachers viewed tobacco use as a habit or lifestyle choice amenable to admonitions about health risks and instructional intervention. Until it was understood to be a serious addiction, with both physiological and social dimensions in its formation and continued reinforcement, and managed as a chronic disease with both behavioral and environmental determinants, rates of tobacco use continued to increase (Green, Eriksen, Bailey, & Husten, 2000). A more systematic approach within primary care settings contributed to progress in smoking cessation. This review, however, will look beyond the clinical setting for clues to the success of smoking prevention that might be emulated in supporting programs and policies in child abuse prevention.

Examples of Effective Use of Community, Statewide, and Media Interventions

Data in support of "best practices" in tobacco control outside the clinical setting come largely from non-experimental, or quasi-experimental, studies of community, statewide, and media interventions. Community interventions usually combine organizational activities or policies in work sites and schools, community-wide policies and programs to limit smoking in public places, and enforcement of laws prohibiting the sale of tobacco to minors. These community efforts have generally been cast within a backdrop of statewide programs, mass media, tax policy, and financial and technical support to local programs. A distinction can be made, then, between community interventions, interventions in communities, and interventions in support of community interventions. Local health departments, with or without the support of a coalition, have typically mounted the community interventions. Nongovernmental organizations have more typically introduced, sponsored, or implemented the interventions in schools, work sites and other community settings. State, federal, and national voluntary health organizations have most typically provided or advocated for the backdrop of statewide, regional or national mass media, tax policy, and grants for financial or technical support of community programs.

Because these broader programs are implemented in complex combinations, evaluation data from controlled community research trials has had to be pieced together. Evidence from selected controlled trials has been combined with data from the 50 state programs, the 10 provincial programs in Canada, and the various state and national programs in smaller countries. A clear pattern emerges over time across the jurisdictions as their programs take distinguishable forms and their smoking rates diverge.

Examples of the Effective Use of Policy for Tobacco Control

The field of tobacco control has worked to incorporate policy–and regulation as an expression of that policy–as a critical component of health promoting initiatives. When dealing with a legal, but addictive product such as tobacco, regulation can be applied at four levels: regulation of the product, of the industry, of community and specific settings within communities, and of the individual. Regulation of products and industry has less relevance to child abuse prevention and accounts for a small proportion of the reduction in tobacco use. However, lessons could be learned from regulation in community settings and at the individual level.

Advertising, sponsorships, and promotion. To change or denormalize the social norm regarding the acceptability of tobacco use and to prevent misleading social cues about tobacco use, a number of countries ban direct and indirect tobacco advertising and others restrict advertising and promotion to some degree. Intensive "counter-marketing" campaigns have been launched to deglamorize smoking.

Smoke-free environments. To protect the public from the hazards of second-hand smoke, most governments limit smoking in public places. Laws that prohibit smoking also have the effect of denormalizing the acceptability of smoking. The notion of denormalizing a behavior has particular relevance to the efforts in child abuse prevention because of historical customs and norms of child discipline and control by parents, guardians, and caretakers. Laws against corporal punishment in schools have possibly had a similar denormalizing value in child abuse prevention.

Taxation. Economic analyses demonstrate that increasing cigarette taxes results in higher quit rates for pregnant women. Higher taxes also prevent or delay relapse during the postpartum period (Coleman, Grossman, & Joyce, 2002).

THE MOTOR VEHICLE SAFETY EXPERIENCE

Although the number of miles traveled is 10 times greater now than in the 1920s, the annual death rate from motor vehicle crashes has decreased 90% (CDC, 1999b). The Institute of Medicine (IOM) estimated that if the mileage death rate of 1972 prevailed in 1996, the number of deaths would have been almost 110,000 instead of the 43,399 that occurred (Bonnie, Fulco, & Liverman, 1999). Between 1970 and 2003, motor vehicle death rates were reduced by half, from a high of almost 30/100,000 population to 14.8/100,000 (MacKenzie, 2000; NHTSA, 2005).

An Epidemiological Approach

In 1966, when William Haddon became the first director of what is now the National Highway Traffic Safety Administration (NHTSA), the field of injury control was in its infancy. Dr. Haddon's most recognized contribution was his analysis of injuries as a function of the host (driver and occupants), agent (vehicle), and environment (roadways), and a time sequence–pre-event (before the crash), event (during the crash), and post-event (after the crash). This analysis of the problem led to an expanded wide array of preventive interventions, many of which contributed to the reduction in motor vehicle fatalities. Modifications to roadways and vehicles, increased use of restraint devices, and decreased rates of drunk driving are the most frequently mentioned reasons explaining the sharp decline in motor vehicle fatality rates (Graham, 1993; Nichols, 1994; Waller, 2001). Changes in individual behavior are frequently cited as significant contributors to the reduction in motor vehicle fatality rates; specifically, increased use of auto restraint devices for adults and children and the reduction in drunk driving. For example, NHTSA (2005) reports the proportion of motor vehicle fatalities that are alcohol-related decreased from 57% in 1982 to 34% in 2003.

How Changes Occurred

The IOM Report, *Reducing the Burden of Injury* (Bonnie et al., 1999) and the CDC, *Ten Great Public Health Achievements* (CDC, 1999a) suggest that the comprehensive, multidisciplinary approach taken to addressing the motor vehicle injury problem is responsible for the successes that have been achieved. This approach requires a sustained commitment to scientific research, government leadership, and public support.

Surveillance systems and research initiatives have provided new knowledge about risk factors and effective interventions. Evidence supports occupant protection and reducing drinking and driving as best practice strategies to prevent motor vehicle injuries (Rivara & MacKenzie, 1999; U.S. Preventive Services Task Force, 1996; Zaza, Thompson, & Harris, 2001).

Government leadership. Many policies related to motor vehicle injuries are determined at the state and local levels, including requirements for using safety equipment (restraints, helmets), driver education and licensing requirements, DUI/DWI standards and penalties. The federal government has provided leadership in reducing some of the disparities through incentive programs whereby states receive reduced federal funding, unless they pass certain laws. States have been able to use federal "402 funding" to evaluate motorcycle helmet laws and implement innovative programs to increase the use of seat belts and child safety seats (Bonnie et al., 1999).

Public support and advocacy. As with tobacco control, the "auto-safety crusade" has adversarial and political roots at the core of the improvements in motor vehicle safety that accrued during the latter half of the 20th century (Isaacs & Schroeder, 2001). The American Medical Association and the American College of Surgeons urged Congress to require that motor vehicles be designed for better safety and Ralph Nader rallied citizen support for the legislation which led to the many safety improvements in vehicles and roadways.

Despite this auspicious beginning, it would be many years before seat belt use would be the rule rather than the exception and airbags would be standard equipment. Graham (1993) identified an important lesson: an excessively adversarial relationship between the public and private sectors retarded progress. While acrimonious debates focused on voluntary vs. mandatory seat belt use, and on active (manual seat belts) vs. passive (air bags and other automatic restraints) protection, little progress was made.

Large-scale federal education programs directed toward state and local safety officials and the general public raised awareness, but achieved modest increases in voluntary seat belt use from 11% in 1980 to 15% in 1984 (Nichols, 1994). However, public information campaigns in several states that promoted public support for mandatory use laws resulted in changed individual behaviors and increased public support for mandatory seat belt laws. Nichols (1994) notes that such public information and education efforts are important elements of programs to change individual safety behavior and necessary to change attitudes, for example, to prepare individuals for legislation. Today the public is well aware of the benefits of safety belts (Girasek & Gielen, 2001).

As with seat belts, use of child restraint devices initially was stimulated by a visible champion, although with far less controversy and a much shorter time frame. In 1978, Dr. Robert Sanders succeeded in getting Tennessee to pass the first law requiring use of car safety seats (Graham, 1993). By 1985 all 50 states (and the District of Columbia) had laws requiring the use of car safety seats (Nichols, 1994). Today's high rates of car seat use are testimony to the fact that a new social norm has been established and the safe transport of children is the expected behavior (Schieber, Gilchrist, & Sleet, 2000).

Changed social norms are most notable in the area of drunk driving. Again, there were champions and a strong grass-roots movement. After drunk driving crashes that killed their daughters, Doris Aiken founded Remove Intoxicated Drivers (RID) and Candy Lightner started Mothers Against Drunk Driving (MADD) (Isaacs & Schroeder, 2001). The IOM Report notes that by elevating the visibility of the families of victims and influencing the public agenda, these groups were able to bring pressure to bear on policymakers (Bonnie et al., 1999). Between 1981 and 1985 state legislatures passed 478 laws to deter drunk driving (Isaacs & Schroeder). In 1984, Congress required states to pass the minimum drinking age of 21 or risk losing a portion of their federal highway safety funds. More recently, Congress used the same approach to encourage states to lower their blood alcohol levels for drunk driving from 0.10 to 0.08.

Public opinions about drinking and driving have changed dramatically. For example, just a quarter century ago, drunk driving was considered a "folk crime," almost a rite of passage for young men (Waller, 2001). Today even the liquor and beer industry promote the idea of having a designated driver (Isaacs & Schroeder, 2001). In a relatively short time, "changes in social norms, in part spurred by such citizen activist groups as MADD, have apparently achieved what many traffic safety professionals believed was virtually impossible: a meaningful change in driver attitudes and behaviors resulting in a reduction of traffic fatalities"(Graham, 1993, p. 524). The motor vehicle safety experience demonstrates how efforts of an active and engaged public can promote significant and sustained changes in both public policy and personal safety behavior.

THE CHILD ABUSE PREVENTION EXPERIENCE

Scarcely a year after Dr. Henry Kempe published his description of the battered child syndrome, the Children's Bureau and American Humane Association had developed a model law for mandatory reporting of child abuse (Kempe, Silverman, Steele, Droegemueller, & Silver, 1962). By 1967, every state had enacted laws requiring health professionals and others to report suspected abuse and neglect. The intent of mandatory reporting laws was to identify previously undetected cases of child maltreatment and protect children from further serious harm by providing families with appropriate services (Chalk & King, 1998). Reporting also provided the beginning of systematic surveillance, enabling public health planning and evaluation in relation to child abuse.

In 1972, Prevent Child Abuse America (PCA America), formerly the National Committee to Prevent Child Abuse, was founded in Chicago. This national organization, with 40 state chapters, is dedicated to preventing child abuse in all its forms. PCA America has taken the lead in raising awareness and changing public attitudes toward child abuse.

We will never know the extent of child maltreatment before reliable statistics were available, but we know it was vastly underestimated. In the early 1960s, the American Humane Association estimated 10,000 cases of child abuse occurred each year, with only 1% of those coming to the attention of the proper authorities (DeFrancis, 1963). Only the most serious cases were reported because most people, even physicians, could not believe parents would hurt their own children (Sanders, 1972).

Efforts to identify, report and investigate suspected cases of child maltreatment have made great strides. Each year, over 3 million children are reported to Child Protective Services (CPS) and about 1 million cases are confirmed. Unfortunately, not enough is being done to prevent child maltreatment and each day three children die of abuse and neglect. Mandatory reporting of child maltreatment is accomplishing what surveillance of tobacco consumption and motor vehicle injuries and deaths accomplished in those fields, except that uniformity of reporting is more difficult in child abuse surveillance.

Public health professionals have recognized child abuse as a public health issue for over 30 years (Hanlon, 1974). In 1984, Surgeon General Koop declared violence as much a public health problem for America as smallpox, polio, TB, and syphilis (Henig, 1997). Ten years later, David Satcher, director of CDC, called violence, including child abuse, the number one public health problem (Applebome, 1993).

More commonly, however, child abuse has been viewed as a social welfare problem or juvenile justice issue. Although this orientation has led to increased detection and improved treatment, it has not prevented child maltreatment from occurring in the first place. Lessons learned from public health and health promotion successes could be helpful in casting child abuse prevention in a primary prevention rather than secondary prevention light.

SPECIFIC LESSONS FOR CHILD ABUSE PREVENTION

Besides the foregoing generalizations that can be drawn from the successes of tobacco control and injury control, the following lessons with more specific implications for prevention of child abuse and neglect are offered.

Lesson 1: Investigate Varied Logic Models or Conceptual Frameworks to Identify New Opportunities for Effective Intervention

Haddon's epidemiological model of host, agent, and environment, in relation to the time sequence, was a conceptual breakthrough for preventing motor vehicle fatalities. A critical examination of existing frameworks in primary prevention could lead to comprehensive theories of change, and suggest how conventional components of public awareness, social services and legal remedies can interface with newer approaches of home visiting and other universal and targeted community-based interventions.

A paradigm shift in primary prevention of child abuse came in 1991 when the U.S. Advisory Board on Child Abuse and Neglect recommended a universal system of voluntary newborn home visitation. Offering some level of home visiting to all families could avoid stigma by reaching mainstream families, while providing more intensive services for at-risk families (Krugman, 1993). The National Research Council and IOM more cautiously recommended home visitation, as part of a comprehensive prevention strategy for preventing child maltreatment, particularly for first-time parents living in high-risk social settings (Chalk & King, 1998).

Responding to the Advisory Board's recommendations, PCA America launched Healthy Families America® (HFA) in 1992. The HFA model is based on 12 "Critical Elements," culled from research findings, evaluations of home visiting programs, and other available evidence. In the first 10 years, HFA grew to over 400 program sites in nearly every state. Other home visiting programs proliferated during the '90s, as well (Schorr, 1997).

After careful review of evidence from 21 studies, the Task Force on Community Preventive Services concluded that home visitation had prevented child maltreatment among high-risk populations by 39% (Bilukha et al., 2005). Home visiting certainly is a positive first step, but important questions about home visiting remain (Gomby, Culross, & Behrman, 1999). How many home visits and what level of intensity are needed to be effective? When should home visiting begin and when is it too late? What curricula work best and under what circumstances? Does focusing on family well-being enhance or dilute efforts to prevent child maltreatment? Very similar questions had to be researched in the smoking cessation literature with respect to optimum timing, numbers and intensity of contacts, and content of the cessation counseling and follow-up.

Home visiting has unique features that are especially important in serving isolated, hard-to-reach families, however, some believe home visiting is necessary, but not sufficient (Weiss, 1993). If home visiting is part of a comprehensive approach to preventing child maltreatment, what else could or should be included, and how should other components be coordinated with home visitation?

Lesson 2: Use a Multi-Disciplinary, Multi-Sector Approach

Community interventions, media advocacy, public information campaigns and legislation combined to reduce tobacco use and improve motor vehicle safety. The child abuse prevention field might be poised to implement lessons from other prevention fields about the advantages of multi-disciplinary and multi-sector approaches. Ramey and Ramey (1993) suggest that achieving robust and lasting effects requires a multi-dimensional approach, addressing multiple domains. The home visiting program itself does not need to be comprehensive, but it should be an integral part of a comprehensive family support program and coordinated with community, statewide, and national program and policy components.

Results from a meta-analysis of evaluation outcomes across 56 family support programs, aimed at preventing child abuse, support this view. All programs were designed to prevent child maltreatment and promote family wellness. Some were for families with no evidence of prior maltreatment and others for families in which maltreatment already had occurred. Most programs showed evidence of effectiveness in preventing child maltreatment and promoting family wellness, with an overall effect size of .41. This indicates outcomes for families in the intervention groups were greater than outcomes for two-thirds of those in the comparison groups (MacLeod & Nelson, 2000). In general, programs for at-risk families were more effective for families with infants, compared to families with older children. Unless families already had experienced child maltreatment, improvements tended to last over time and even increase.

Multi-component programs used a multidisciplinary and multi-sector approach; whereas home visiting programs did not. Multi-component programs were more comprehensive. In multi-component programs, the home visiting component was broadened to encompass home management, personal development of the mother, and linkages to government and community resources. Community development and separate child-care and/or preschool education were additional components. Services were provided in different locations and families had contact with several individuals, instead of one home visitor.

Multi-component programs were more effective overall than home visiting only programs. Multi-component programs were equally effective serving low-income families or a mix of moderate and low-income families; whereas, home visiting programs were effective for a mix of moderate and low-income families. Differences in the two approaches might account for different outcomes.

If multi-component programs are more effective than home visiting only programs, how should policymakers and community leaders proceed? How can they add components, such as concrete and social support, community development and child care? Evidence suggests they should not expect home visiting programs to do everything. In fact, home visiting programs were less effective when too many components were added to the tasks of the home visitor (MacLeod & Nelson, 2000). It would be better to involve other sectors of the community.

Compared with the control group, measures of family well-being were significantly better for families enrolled in the home visiting program. Less than 1.5% of families in the home-visited group had substantiated child maltreatment (Galano et al., 2001). Families in the control group also had comparatively low rates, perhaps because they benefited from other services in the community. Increased surveillance by home visitors also might have obscured differences between the groups.

Lesson 3: Normalize Desired Behaviors and Denormalize Undesirable Behaviors

Laws that mandate behavior, coupled with efforts to facilitate behavioral change, are a powerful combination to establish new social norms, as shown by the tobacco and motor vehicle injury experiences. This combination also changed behaviors of professionals in reporting child abuse. Laws requiring professionals and others to report suspected child maltreatment and the data that flowed from compliance with those laws set new societal expectations. Assuring confidentiality of the reporter and setting the threshold at suspected maltreatment, offered protection and made reporting behaviors easier to adopt.

Changing public behavior of parents seems to work in a similar fashion. Reduced rates of smoking in public places and high rates of car safety seat use demonstrate new social norms. Laws in 50 states demonstrate society's expectation that nonsmokers are to be protected from secondhand smoke, that children are to be transported safely, and that people should not be exposed to the risk of drunk drivers on their roads (Zwerling & Jones, 1999).

Legislation spurred professionals to adopt a new social norm about reporting child maltreatment, curtailed smoking in public places, and caused parents to use child safety seats. Laws requiring all parents to participate in home visiting, however, would be viewed as inappropriate. Fortunately, health-related social norms can change without legal mandates. Recall examples of adopting family planning methods in the early decades of the last century, formula-feeding infants in the '40s, immunizing against polio in the '50s (though school entry laws later solidified this behavior), changing childbirth practices in the '70s, and positioning infants on their back to sleep in the '90s. Whether consumer-driven or instigated by professionals, these examples of widespread change occurred because caring for children is a core value. Families overcame inertia, fear, and inconvenience after becoming convinced that the new approach would benefit their child (even though formula-feeding later proved to be less beneficial than breastfeeding).

Supporting parents of newborns could become a social norm. Offering support to all parents sends a message that parents deserve support because they are parents, not because they are problems. When offering and accepting support is normalized, at-risk parents will be more inclined to participate in home visiting and/or other programs. It is what parents do, if they want to be the best parents for their child.

Lesson 4: Balance Efficacy, Feasibility, and Cultural Appropriateness

Balancing efficacy and feasibility starts with requiring standards to be evidence-based, and not imposing standards until sufficient evidence is available. Variation occurred when states and local jurisdictions purposefully set their own motor vehicle safety standards. This led to innovations that later could be phased in, using incentives and special grants. Feasibility could be determined in different settings and realistic expectations set before requiring every state to adopt new standards or laws. Moreover, "experts" are not always correct, even when they are in positions of authority. For years, health professionals urged parents to put babies to sleep on their stomach, never on their back. Recommended practice became conventional wisdom without ever questioning underlying assumptions. Thanks to pediatricians in Australia, we now know babies need to sleep on their back to prevent Sudden Infant Death Syndrome (SIDS).

HFA and other national home visiting programs admirably seek to reach more at-risk families in diverse communities, without jeopardizing quality or diluting effectiveness. However, requiring adherence to excessively precise process measures may prove to be a misguided attempt to control quality at the expense of needed adaptation to local culture and circumstances. For example, codifying 12 Critical Elements into 144 credentialing standards and requiring HFA programs to demonstrate adherence to each of these standards could unnecessarily restrain professional discretion, innovation and adaptation, and result in an overly regimented, stultified service strategy that can no longer respond to family needs. Other home visiting programs follow strict replication models, with little room for flexibility.

This approach is problematic because some standards have insufficient evidence to support them, while many are not linked to outcome measures. Moreover, available evidence is not always reflected in existing standards or used to develop new standards. Striving to meet overly stringent standards can be counterproductive when it dampens innovation and stifles development of new knowledge. Premature closure on defining best practice impedes discovery of more effective interventions. Searching for and discovering the optimal level and content of smoking cessation for physicians to impart within their crowded clinical encounters has led to highly efficient medical record reminders and brief physician prompts and queries of their patients.

Planned innovation could provide much-needed knowledge based on experience. For example, if programs could temporarily ignore selected credentialing standards and purposefully adjust the frequency of home visits to meet families' needs, researchers and practitioners might discover that families participate in home visiting longer and achieve better outcomes.

CONCLUSIONS

This analysis raises, in particular, the question of how to frame the child abuse prevention issue so it can benefit from some of the lessons of tobacco control and motor vehicle control campaigns and politics. The tobacco industry is a specific villain to chase and curtail in its business practices, if not put out of business. The automobile industry also provided a specific villain during a crucial phase of the injury control campaigns. These industry targets helped to galvanize the public against greedy corporate enemies of health and human, especially child, welfare. Child abuse has no corporate enemy to blame. Blaming the parents, who perpetrate child abuse, can be counterproductive by driving them further underground and away from effective treatment and prevention services and programs. Although sexual abuse is not the focus of this paper, it serves to illustrate one approach to framing the issue. Policies to protect children from possible exposure to sexual offenders and media campaigns to warn the general public could prove more beneficial than putting the full responsibility on the shoulders of health professionals (U.S. General Accounting Office, 1996).

By concentrating the burden on a few identifiable entities (tobacco companies, automobile industry, and child molesters) and dispersing the benefactors (all children), as with most consumer protection regulations, society has greater incentive to mobilize and influence policy. Conversely, when blame is dispersed to many, and benefits are concentrated on a few, there is little incentive to mobilize. John Q. Wilson refers to Entrepreneurial Politics, in which effective action usually requires skillful use of the media to generate public support or outrage, as Ralph Nader did with auto industries (Schlozman & Tierney, 1986).

Policy strategies for home visiting or other child abuse prevention programs will depend upon how the initiative is framed. If it is viewed as a program for a few high-risk families, funded primarily by tax dollars, the benefits are concentrated on a few and the costs or burdens are distributed to the general public. This is termed *Client Politics*. It is common to programs run by social service or other organizations when government agencies provide funding for programs such as CPS and maternal child health programs.

However, if home visiting is viewed as a supportive service for all parents, funded by insurance or tax dollars, both benefits and costs or burdens are distributed. When large numbers of people benefit and costs are borne by most of society (Wilson's Majoritarian Politics), major political parties usually get involved. The public often weighs in because everyone stands to gain and/or lose when decisions are made about social security, education and homeland defense.

Child abuse prevention programs should strive to avoid what Wilson terms Interest Group Politics, where benefits are concentrated on one identifiable group and costs are concentrated on another identifiable group. Opposing groups have strong incentives to affect the outcome when resources are limited in a zero-sum game, where one gains and the other loses, but the general public is usually unaware of or uninterested in the issue. One of the lessons from traffic safety is that struggles among interest groups (insurers, automobile manufacturers, consumer advocates, and government officials) retarded progress. The tobacco wars stalled in legislation when the advocacy groups disagreed, among other things, on the extent of punishment and financial burden to be heaped on the tobacco industry. Advocates for home visiting programs and other preventive initiatives could be effective if they work together and find common ground.

Other conclusions of this analysis are reflected in the generalizations and lessons drawn from the tobacco control and motor vehicle injury control experiences. Those conclusions depend to a large degree on the political framing of the issue in broader policy debates.

REFERENCES

Applebome, P. (1993, September 26). CDC's new chief worries as much about bullets as about bacteria. *New York Times*, p. A7.

Bilukha, O., Hahn, R., Crosby, A., Fullilove, M., Liberman, A., Moscicki, E. et al. (2005). The effectiveness of early childhood home visitation in preventing violence: A systematic review. *American Journal of Preventive Medicine, 28*(Suppl. 1), 11-39.

Bonnie, R., Fulco, C., & Liverman, C. (Eds.) (1999). *Reducing the burden of injury, advancing prevention and treatment.* Institute of Medicine, Washington, DC: National Academy Press.

Centers for Disease Control and Prevention (1999a). Ten great public health achievements–United States, 1900-1999. *Morbidity and Mortality Weekly Report, 48*, 241-243.

Centers for Disease Control and Prevention (1999b). Motor vehicle safety: A 20th century public health achievement. *Morbidity and Mortality Weekly Report, 48*, 369-374.

Chalk, R., & King, P. (Eds.) (1998). *Violence in families: Assessing prevention and treatment programs* (pp. 7-8, 161). Washington, DC: Institute of Medicine.

Colman, G., Grossman, M., & Joyce, T. (2002). *The effect of cigarette excise taxes on smoking before, during and after pregnancy* (No. 9245). Cambridge, MA: National Bureau of Economic Research.

DeFrancis, V. (1963). *Child abuse.* Denver, CO: American Humane Association.

Girasek, D., & Gielen, A. (2003). The effectiveness of injury prevention strategies: What does the public believe? *Health Education and Behavior, 30*, 287-304.

Gomby, D., Culross, P., & Behrman, R. (1999). Home visiting: Recent program evaluations–analysis and recommendations. *The Future of Children, 9*, 4-24.

Graham, J. (1993). Injuries from traffic crashes: Meeting the challenge. *Annual Review of Public Health, 14*, 515-543.

Green, L. (2001). From research to "best practices" in other settings and populations. *American Journal of Health Behavior, 25*, 165-178.

Green, L., Eriksen, M., Bailey, L., & Husten, C. (2000). Achieving the implausible in the next decade: Tobacco control objectives. *American Journal of Public Health, 90*, 337-339.

Hanlon, J. (1974). *Public health administration and practice* (6th ed.). St. Louis, MO: CV Mosby Co.

Henig, R. (1997). *The people's health: A memoir of public health and its evolution at Harvard.* Washington, DC: Joseph Henry Press.

Isaacs, S., & Schroeder, S. (2001, June 4). Where the public good prevailed. *The American Prospect, 12,* 1-10.

Kempe, C., Silverman, F., Steele, B., Droegemueller, W., & Silver, H. (1962). The battered child syndrome. *Journal of the American Medical Association, 181,* 17-24.

Krugman, R. (1993). Universal home visiting: Recommendation from the US Advisory Board on Child Abuse and Neglect. *The Future of Children, 3*(3), 184-191.

Lancaster, B. (1992). Closing the gap between research and practice. *Health Education Quarterly, 19,* 408-411.

MacKenzie, E. (2000). Epidemiology of injuries: Current trends and future challenges. *Epidemiologic Reviews, 22,* 112-119.

MacLeod, J., & Nelson, G. (2000). Programs for the promotion of family wellness and the prevention of child maltreatment: A meta-analytic review. *Child Abuse and Neglect, 24,* 1127-1149.

National Highway Traffic Safety Administration (2005). *State alcohol related fatality rates 2003* (No. DOT HS 809 830). Washington, DC: U.S. Department of Transportation.

Nichols, J. (1994). Changing public behavior for better health: Is education enough? *American Journal of Preventive Medicine, 10* (Suppl. 1), 19-22.

Ramey, C., & Ramey, S. (1993). Home visiting programs and the health and development of young children. *The Future of Children, 3*(3), 129-139.

Rivara, F., & MacKenzie, E. (1999). Systematic reviews of strategies to prevent motor vehicle injuries. *American Journal of Preventive Medicine, 16*(Suppl. 1), 1-90.

Sanders, R. (1972). Resistance to dealing with parents of battered children. *Pediatrics, 50,* 853.

Schieber, R., Gilchrist, J., & Sleet, D. (2000). Legislative and regulatory strategies to reduce childhood unintentional injuries. *The Future of Children, 10*(1), 111-136.

Schlozman, K., & Tierney, J. (1986). *Organized interests and American democracy.* New York: Harper & Row Publishers, Inc.

Schorr, L. (1997). *Common purpose: Strengthening families and neighborhoods to rebuild America.* New York: Bantam Doubleday Dell Publishing Group, Inc.

U.S. General Accounting Office (1996). *Sex offender treatment: Research results inconclusive about what works to reduce recidivism.* Washington, DC: U.S. General Accounting Office.

U.S. Preventive Services Task Force (1996). *Guide to clinical preventive services* (2nd ed.). Baltimore: Williams and Wilkens.

Waller, P. (2001). Public health's contribution to motor vehicle injury prevention. *American Journal of Preventive Medicine, 21*(Suppl.), 1-2.

Weiss, H. (1993). Home visits: Necessary but not sufficient. *The Future of Children, 3*(3), 113-128.

Zaza, S., Thompson, R., & Harris, K. (Eds.) (2001). The guide to community preventive services, reducing injuries to motor vehicle occupants: Systematic reviews of evidence, recommendations from the Task Force on Community Preventive

Services, and expert commentary. *American Journal of Preventive Medicine, 21*(Suppl.), 1-90.

Zwerling, C., & Jones, M. (1999). Evaluation of the effectiveness of low blood alcohol concentration laws for younger drivers. *American Journal of Preventive Medicine, 16*(Suppl. 1), 76-8.

doi:10.1300/J005v34n01_10

Index

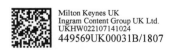